The Complete
Whole Body Reset
Cookbook

Healthy Whole Body Reset Recipes and Rigorous

4-Week Diet Plan to Boost Your Metabolism

Latoya Limon

Table of Contents

The Whole Body Reset diet is a three-phase plan lasting for 15 days that involves consuming low-calorie smoothies and gradually reintroducing solid food. During the initial phase, smoothies in white, red, and green varieties are the only source of nutrition for breakfast, lunch, and dinner. In the second phase, two smoothies are consumed daily alongside a solid meal, such as a salad, sandwich, or stir-fry. In the final phase, one smoothie is replaced with another solid meal. The Whole Body Reset diet is vegan and vegetarian-friendly, gluten-free friendly, halal-friendly, and kosher-friendly, making it accessible to a wide range of dietary preferences and restrictions.

In addition to the dietary guidelines, the program also includes recommendations for exercise. Walking at least 12,000 steps per day is encouraged, as well as resistance training for at least five minutes, five days per week. The exercises recommended by the program include the reverse fly, dips, planks, and hamstring curls. The Whole Body Reset trains the body to use energy more efficiently and burn calories faster, leading to sustainable weight loss and improved overall health.

Fundamentals of Whole Body Reset

What Is Whole Body Reset?

The Whole Body Reset diet is based on the concept that a low-calorie, plant-based diet mainly consisting of smoothies for 15 days can teach the body to utilize energy more efficiently and burn calories faster, even during sleep. The Whole Body Reset diet can facilitate sustainable and long-term weight loss when combined with resistance exercise three days per week.

- The recipes are adaptable for a vegan or vegetarian diet.
- The recipes can be modified to adhere to a gluten-free diet.
- The recipes can be adapted to follow a Halal diet.
- The recipes can be modified to comply with a Kosher diet.

The Whole Body Reset diet is a 15-day program designed to reset the body by replacing solid foods with smoothies for the first five days, gradually reintroducing solid food, and focusing on plant-based, low-calorie meals. Here are the fundamentals of the diet:

Three Phases: The diet has three phases, each lasting five days. In the first phase, smoothies are the sole source of nutrition, with white, red, and green varieties for breakfast, lunch, and dinner. In the second phase, two smoothies and one solid meal are consumed daily, and in the

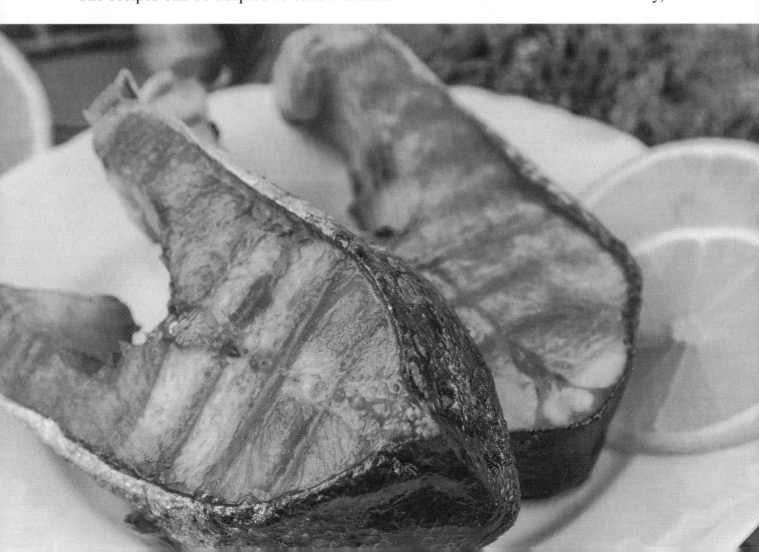

third phase, one smoothie is replaced with another solid meal.

Plant-based, Low-calorie Meals: The Whole Body Reset diet is primarily plant-based, emphasizing fruits and vegetables. It is also low in calories, with each smoothie containing approximately 270 to 325 calories.

Exercise: Exercise is a crucial component of the Whole Body Reset diet. The diet creator, Harley Pasternak, recommends walking at least 12,000 steps per day, which can be achieved by making small changes in daily routines. Resistance exercises, such as the reverse fly, dips, planks, and hamstring curls, are also recommended.

Modifications for Special Diets: The diet is vegan, vegetarian, gluten-free, halal, and kosher-friendly, with recipes that can be easily modified to fit different dietary needs.

Rapid Weight Loss: The Whole Body Reset diet is designed for rapid weight loss, with calorie restriction and increased physical activity as the primary drivers. However, it is essential to consult a healthcare provider before starting any new diet or exercise program.

"Lose Weight with the Body Reset Diet? „

Following the Whole Body Reset diet is likely to result in weight loss since the smoothies are low in calories and packed with fruits and vegetables, which can create a calorie deficit. However, there is no clinical evidence supporting this diet's effectiveness in the long term. Maintaining the weight loss achieved during the initial deprivation period also depends on the types of solid foods reintroduced after the initial 15-day period.

The Whole Body Reset diet aligns with vegetarianism, linked to consuming fewer calories, weighing less, and having better overall health. This diet encourages the consumption of whole fruits and vegetables, a healthier alternative to ultra-processed and refined foods. Rapid weight loss in the initial phase of this diet may also motivate some individuals to continue losing weight.

The Whole Body Reset diet can lead to short-term weight loss due to significantly reduced calorie intake for over two weeks. However, long-term weight loss is uncertain since reintroducing solid foods will increase calorie intake, which may result in regaining the lost weight. As there is no research on the long-term outcomes of this diet, strategies for weight-loss management have not been clearly defined. It is also important to note that this diet is designed to be short-term and is not intended as a long-term solution for weight management.

"How Does This Diet Work? „

- Consume three smoothies daily during the first 5 days, each containing approximately 270 to 325 calories.
- On days 6 through 10, substitute one smoothie with a solid meal, such as a salad or vegetable stir-fry.
- During days 11 through 15, replace two smoothies with solid meals.

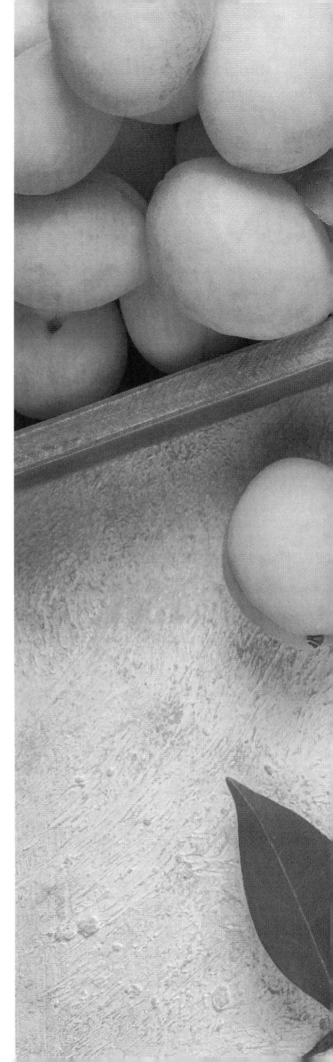

• Use "The Body Reset Diet" cookbook.

The Whole Body Reset diet is designed to quickly reset your eating habits by substituting solid foods with nutritious, low-calorie, plant-based smoothies. According to Gaby Vaca-Flores, a registered dietitian and the founder of Glow+Greens, a nutrition and skin care consultancy based in Santa Monica, California, the creator of The Whole Body Reset diet devised this dietary pattern for individuals seeking rapid weight loss. "Calorie restriction and increased physical activity lead to rapid weight loss," she explains.

You'll have three smoothies and two snacks daily during the first five days of the Body Reset Diet. These smoothies come in three varieties:

• White smoothies contain milk or Greek yogurt and provide a good source of protein.

• Red smoothies are full of fruits that give you energy.

• Green smoothies consist of vegetables to keep you feeling full at night.

In addition to following the diet, the creator of the Body Reset Diet, Harley Pasternak, encourages exercise. Rather than going to the gym daily, Pasternak suggests walking at least 12,000 steps daily, which can be achieved by making small changes in your daily routine, such as getting off the bus or train one stop early or taking the stairs instead of the elevator. Pasternak also recommends resistance exercise for at least five minutes five days per week or light resistance training for five minutes three times weekly. These exercises, such as reverse fly, dips, planks, and hamstring curls, help build muscle and may prevent arthritis, diabetes, obesity, and other health issues. The Whole Body Reset diet book provides full instructions for each exercise, and beginners can complete the circuit once, intermediates twice, and gym veterans three times.

" The Advantages of the Whole Body Reset Diet „

The Whole Body Reset diet, also known as the Body Reset diet, is a low-calorie, plant-based diet that primarily consists of smoothies. This diet has several potential advantages, including:

Weight Loss: The Whole Body Reset diet promotes weight loss by reducing calorie intake and increasing energy expenditure. The diet is low in calories but high in nutrients, which can help keep you full and satisfied while consuming fewer calories.

Improved Nutrient Intake: The smoothies in The Whole Body Reset diet are made from whole foods such as fruits, vegetables, and nuts, which are rich in vitamins, minerals, and other essential nutrients. You can improve your overall nutrient intake and support optimal health by consuming smoothies made from these nutrient-dense foods.

Increased Energy: The Whole Body Reset diet is designed to train your body to use energy more efficiently, which can lead to increased energy levels throughout the day. By consuming nutrient-dense smoothies, your body can access a steady stream of energy to help you feel more alert and focused.

Reduced Inflammation: The Whole Body Reset diet is rich in anti-inflammatory foods such as fruits and vegetables, which can help reduce inflammation. Chronic inflammation has been linked to numerous health problems, including heart disease, diabetes, and cancer.

Improved Digestion: The high fiber content of the smoothies in The Whole Body Reset diet can help to improve digestion and promote regular bowel movements. By consuming a fiber-rich diet, you can also support a healthy gut

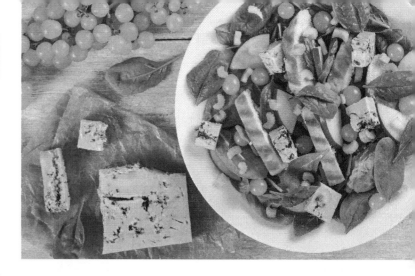

microbiome linked to numerous health benefits. Overall, the Whole Body Reset diet can effectively kickstart weight loss and improve overall health. However, consulting a healthcare professional before starting any new diet or exercise program is essential.

"Who Should Not Try the Body Reset Diet? „

The Whole Body Reset diet is not recommended for individuals with an eating disorder or those in recovery from one. People with diabetes or heart disease should consult a healthcare provider or registered dietitian before starting the diet.

According to Pumper, The Whole Body Reset diet is designed for those who desire rapid weight loss, but caution is required due to adverse effects. The plan is regimented and restrictive, leaving little room for flexibility, possibly leading to bingeing. Additionally, the diet's weight loss effects are typically short-lived, and adherence to the plan tends to wane over time, resulting in weight regain.

Vaca-Flores believes that "quick-fix" diets like The Whole Body Reset are unsustainable and may lead to more weight gain. Instead, Pumper suggests cultivating healthy habits and behaviors to help you achieve your goals.

The Whole Body Reset diet is composed of three five-day phases. In Phase I, you will only consume smoothies and snacks. In Phase II, you will add one meal and two daily snacks to the smoothies. In Phase III, you will decrease your smoothie intake to one per day and consume two meals and two snacks. After completing the third phase, you will enter a maintenance phase where you can have two "free" meals per week and eat or drink whatever you want.

This diet emphasizes low-fat foods and healthy fats such as nuts, seeds, and avocado. It also focuses on lean protein, particularly milk protein for the smoothies, and calories from high-fiber carbohydrates, primarily fruits, and vegetables.

Smoothies: The Body Reset program emphasizes smoothies, categorized into three types: white for breakfast, red for lunch, and green for dinner. The basic white smoothie recipe includes an apple, pear, or peach, a banana, a few almonds, milk, yogurt, and spices to taste. Red smoothies consist of berries, half an orange, one scoop of protein powder, and one tablespoon of ground flaxseed. Green smoothies include two cups of greens such as spinach, kale, baby arugula, romaine lettuce, a pear, grapes, Greek yogurt, avocado, and lime juice. The program provides six recipes for each type of smoothie, and substitutions are allowed if desired, such as almonds in place of avocado or tofu instead of Greek yogurt.

Fruits and Vegetables: In the Body Reset diet, opting for fruits and vegetables with higher fiber content, particularly for snacks, is crucial. Additionally, consuming the skin of fruits such as apples and pears instead of peeling them is recommended. Snack options that the diet promotes include apples, pears, and peaches.

Milk and Yogurt: According to Pasternak, dairy products have been unfairly criticized in recent years. He argues that milk has been consumed by humans for centuries and is a good source of protein, calcium, vitamin D, and other essential nutrients. The Whole Body Reset diet includes the following dairy and non-dairy milk products:

Plain nonfat Greek yogurt

Nonfat milk

Non-dairy milk alternatives.

Nuts and Seeds

Almonds

Walnuts

Flaxseeds

Whole Grains

All grain products should be whole grain.

Some examples include:

Popcorn

Whole-grain crackers

Whole wheat tortillas

Whole grain bread

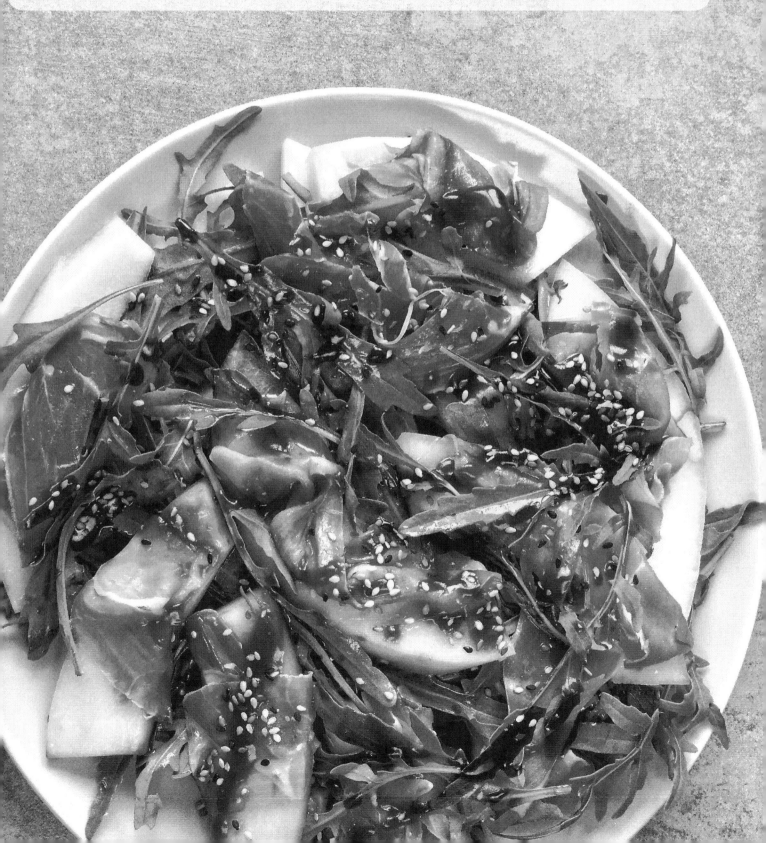

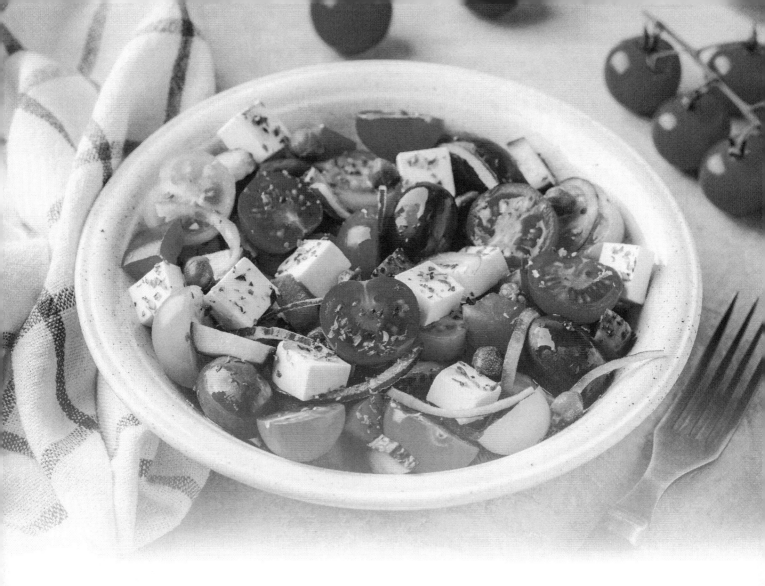

Lean Protein, Meat, and Fish

Choose lean sources of protein, meat, and fish, such as:

Skinless chicken breast

Turkey breast

Lean cuts of beef or pork

Fish (such as salmon, trout, or tilapia)

Tofu or tempeh (for vegetarians/vegans)

"Which Foods Are Not Allowed to Be Eaten?"

The Whole Body Reset diet is a 15-day program to jumpstart weight loss and promote healthier eating habits. The diet emphasizes consuming mostly smoothies and other low-fat, high-fiber foods such as fruits, vegetables, and lean proteins. While there is some flexibility in the diet, several foods are not allowed to be eaten in the Body Reset program.

Processed Food: One of the most notable restrictions in The Whole Body Reset diet is avoiding processed foods. This means that any food that has been heavily processed, such as fast food, frozen dinners, or packaged snacks, is not allowed on a diet. Processed foods are typically high in calories, sodium, and unhealthy fats and can contribute to weight gain and other health problems.

Added Sugar: In addition to processed foods, The Whole Body Reset diet also restricts the consumption of added sugars. Any food or drink with added sugars, such as soda, candy, or baked goods, is prohibited on a diet. Added sugars are a significant contributor to excess calories and can lead to several health problems, including diabetes and obesity.

High-Fat food: Another food group restricted on The Whole Body Reset diet is high-fat foods. While the diet includes some healthy fats in nuts, seeds, and avocado, it restricts the consumption of high-fat foods such as butter, cheese, and fatty meats. These foods are typically high in calories and can contribute to weight gain and other health problems, such as high cholesterol and heart disease.

Alcohol: The Whole Body Reset diet also restricts the consumption of alcohol. While a small amount of alcohol, such as a glass of red wine, may have some health benefits, excessive alcohol consumption can harm health and contribute to weight gain. The diet recommends avoiding alcohol entirely during the 15-day program.

Caffeine: Finally, The Whole Body Reset diet encourages the avoidance of caffeine. While caffeine can provide a temporary energy boost, it can also lead to dehydration, jitteriness, and other adverse side effects. The diet recommends limiting caffeine intake during the 15-day program and suggests switching to decaf coffee or herbal tea.

While several foods are not allowed on the Body Reset diet, the program also has some flexibility. The diet allows for substitutions and encourages the consumption of various fruits, vegetables, and lean proteins. By avoiding processed foods, added sugars, high-fat foods, alcohol, and caffeine, The Whole Body Reset diet can help jumpstart weight loss and promote healthier eating habits.

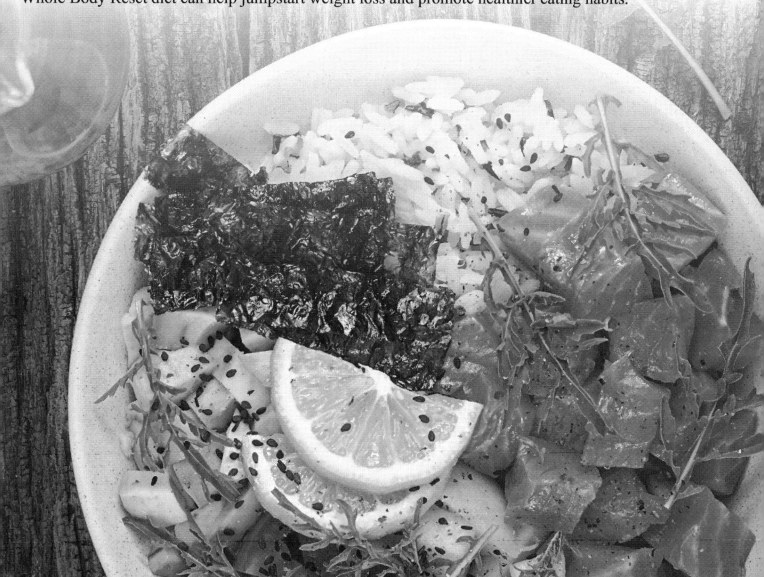

" Doing the Whole Body Reset Diet on A Budget „

According to Pumper, The Whole Body Reset diet is affordable for those on a budget as it requires no signature food products or meal delivery services. Instead, you can use everyday foods found at your local grocery store. To follow this diet on a budget, Pumper suggests several strategies:

• Plan and create a realistic food budget.

• Check what you already have in your pantry, fridge, and freezer to avoid overbuying.

• Look for sales and use coupons to save money.

• Buy the store brand or generic products instead of name brands.

• Shop only once a week with a prepared list of meals and stick to it to avoid overspending.

• Eat a healthy snack or meal before going to the grocery store to prevent impulse buying.

• Buy animal-based and plant-based proteins in bulk and freeze what you do not need.

• Use canned or frozen foods, such as canned chicken, fish, beans, and frozen fruits and vegetables.

• Supplement high-cost meats with lower-cost proteins like beans, lentils, eggs, and low-fat dairy.

• Buy seasonal produce to save money.

"Diet Tips „

1. According to the Body Reset diet, certain foods should be avoided to achieve the best results. While the diet doesn't necessarily restrict any particular food groups, it does emphasize the importance of making good nutritional choices and avoiding processed foods.

2. One of the key features of The Whole Body Reset diet is its focus on consuming smoothies and snacks during the first three phases of the program. Therefore, it's recommended that dieters avoid foods high in calories and low in nutrients during these phases.

3. Processed foods such as chips, cookies, and candy are strictly prohibited, as are sugary drinks and alcoholic beverages. Pasternak also recommends avoiding red meat, processed meats, and fried foods.

4. While dairy products are included in the diet plan, it's recommended to choose low-fat or nonfat options. Additionally, cheese should be limited to no more than one ounce per day.

5. During the first phase of the diet, which involves consuming only smoothies and snacks, avoiding foods not included in the recommended recipes is essential. This means avoiding meals not explicitly designated as an "S-meal" during Phases II and III.

6. Regarding portion sizes, Pasternak recommends keeping meals and snacks small and frequent. The idea is to graze throughout the day to maintain consistent blood sugar levels and reduce hunger.

7. While there aren't any strict rules about which foods to avoid, The Whole Body Reset diet emphasizes the importance of making good nutritional choices and avoiding processed foods. Dieters can achieve better health and weight loss results by focusing on whole, nutrient-dense foods and avoiding high-calorie, low-nutrient options.

" Pros of the Body Reset Diet „

• **Provides ample nutrition through fruits, vegetables, and fiber:** Smoothies are an effective way to incorporate a variety of nutrient-

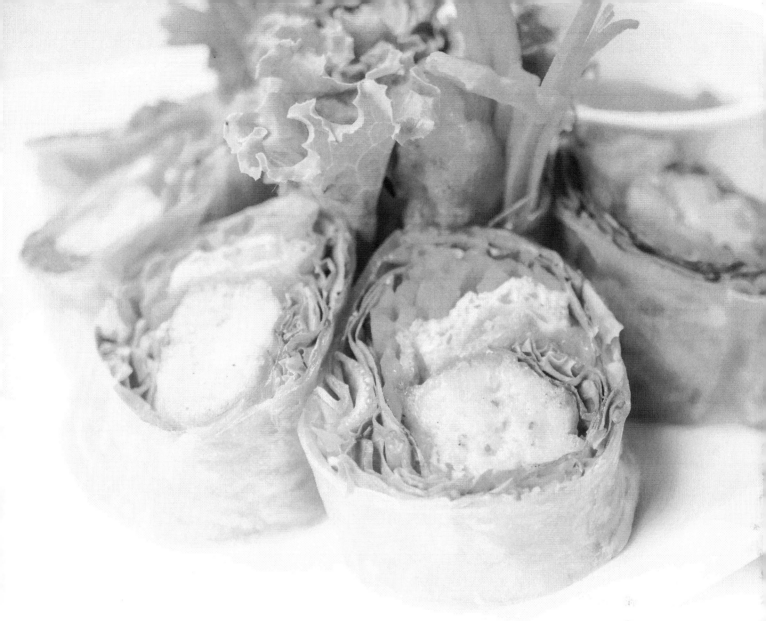

rich fruits and vegetables into your diet while boosting your fiber intake. This can be especially helpful for those who struggle to consume enough produce and fiber on a daily basis.

- **Easy to follow:** The Whole Body Reset diet is relatively straightforward, with minimal calorie-counting involved. Simply follow the program of smoothies, snacks, and meals as outlined in the diet blueprint, which also offers suggestions for keeping snacks around 150 calories each.

- **Includes exercise:** While the diet claims to allow you to "eat more, exercise less," it still calls for a significant amount of physical activity, such as walking a minimum of 10,000 steps per day and incorporating resistance training. Combining dietary changes with exercise is widely recognized as an effective way to promote weight loss and improve overall health.

- **Low-fat, high-fiber:** The Whole Body Reset diet emphasizes the consumption of low-fat foods, such as skim milk and fat-free Greek yogurt. In addition, the diet encourages adequate fiber intake, which is crucial for maintaining healthy digestion and may also help reduce the risk of certain types of cancer.

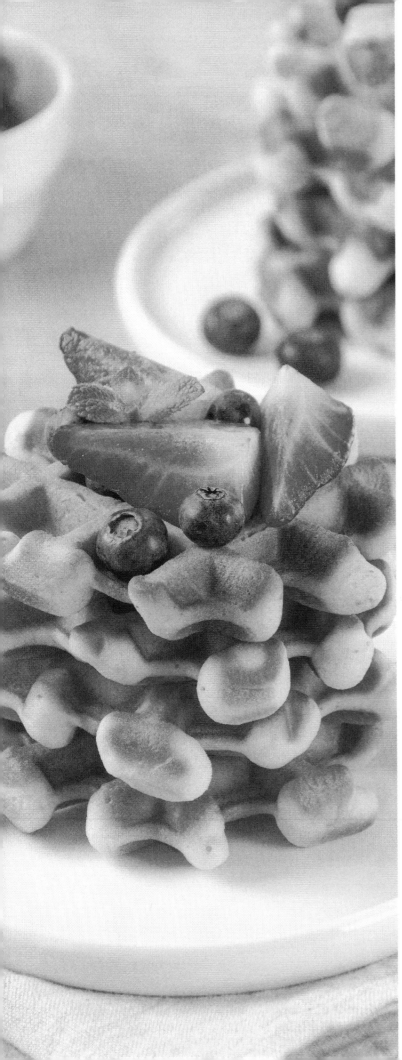

- **Highly restrictive:** The Whole Body Reset diet can leave you feeling very hungry, particularly during the initial five days, as you'll be consuming only three smoothies and two 150-calorie snacks per day, providing fewer than 1,200 calories in total.

- **Time-consuming:** Although making smoothies is not difficult, blending multiple smoothies and cleaning the blender can be time-consuming. Additionally, you'll need to keep the smoothies refrigerated if you don't drink them immediately, which can be inconvenient.

- **Potentially unappetizing:** While The Whole Body Reset diet offers various ingredient and spice options to make the smoothies more palatable, not everyone will enjoy drinking smoothies made with certain ingredients such as Swiss chard and protein powder. To succeed on the Body Reset diet, you'll need to like, or at least tolerate, all the different types of smoothies.

- **Unsustainable:** Although you may lose weight during the 15-day cycle of the Body Reset diet, you may regain some or all of the weight when you go back to your regular diet. Pasternak recommends lifestyle changes and additional "resets" to help maintain weight loss.

- **Limited food groups:** The Whole Body Reset diet emphasizes fruits and vegetables, but may lack whole grains and protein, which are essential components of a balanced diet.

- **Low calorie intake:** The first five days of The Whole Body Reset diet provide fewer than 1,200 calories per day, which is well below the recommended calorie intake of 1,500 calories per day for safe, gradual weight loss. This can lead to hunger and feelings of deprivation.

- **Risk of weight regain:** The weight loss effects

of The Whole Body Reset diet are likely to be short-term, and you may regain weight once you return to your normal eating patterns. The diet's emphasis on quick weight loss can result in a cycle of weight loss and regain, making it challenging to achieve permanent weight loss.

Is the Body Reset Diet Easy to Follow?

Although the Body Reset diet's primary focus is on consuming smoothies, sticking to this diet may be difficult as you might crave solid foods and miss your typical meals. While the crunchy snacks allowed every day can help curb your cravings, you'll need strong willpower to adhere to the Body Reset diet.

The convenience of this diet is subjective. On the one hand, it requires work as you have to prepare your smoothies daily and have your snacks ready to munch on. But it might save you time since you can consume your "meals" quickly or even while on the go.

There are ways to make this diet more efficient, such as preparing all the ingredients for each smoothie in advance and storing them in the freezer in a Ziploc bag, a strategy many dieters use.

During at least the first phase of the Body Reset diet, you may experience hunger. Satiety, the feeling of being satisfied after eating, is essential for your overall health, and smoothies can help you feel full due to their fiber, whole grains, and vegetable content. However, consuming these foods in their whole form might keep you fuller for longer. Additionally, the lack of solid foods during phase one might make it challenging to complete the diet.

If you like smoothies, you'll probably enjoy the taste of the Body Reset diet. A wide range of smoothie recipes is available in "The Body Reset Diet" book, including apple pie smoothie and Caribbean kale smoothie. You're not limited to drinking the same smoothie every day as long as you follow the macronutrient profiles.

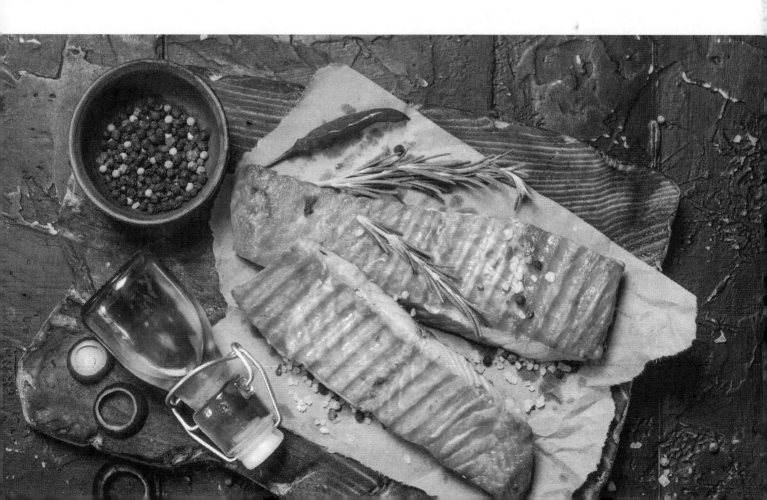

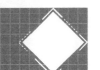

4-Week Meal Plan

Week 1

Day 1:
Breakfast: Spiced Zucchini Strips
Lunch: Herbed Spinach Lasagna
Snack: Delicious Hoisin Button Mushrooms
Dinner: Spicy White Fish and Tomato Soup
Dessert: Prosciutto Wrapped Plums

Day 2:
Breakfast: Sesame Bread
Lunch: Mayo Coleslaw
Snack: Simple Boiled Unshelled Peanuts
Dinner: Avocado-Tuna Stuffed Cucumber Roll
Dessert: Nutty Protein Truffles

Day 3:
Breakfast: Spinach-Grapefruit Pineapple Smoothie
Lunch: Tangy Mushroom Stroganoff
Snack: Spiced Nuts Mix
Dinner: Mustard Chicken Nuggets
Dessert: Strawberry-Applesauce Ice Cream

Day 4:
Breakfast: Chocolate-Blueberry Oatmeal
Lunch: Herbed Veggie Stew
Snack: Nutty Cranberry Oats
Dinner: Chicken Mushroom Meatloaf
Dessert: Butter Apple Pie

Day 5:
Breakfast: Apple Spinach-Curry Crepes
Lunch: Baked Potatoes and Sweet Lentils
Snack: Crispy Flaxseed Crackers
Dinner: Lemony Mustard Pork
Dessert: Simple Whipped Cream

Day 6:
Breakfast: Chocolate Cherry Smoothie
Lunch: Tasty Quinoa and Roasted Vegetables
Snack: Lemony Roasted Chickpeas
Dinner: Garlicky Balsamic Lamb Chops
Dessert: Chocolate Banana Bread

Day 7:
Breakfast: Nutty Chicken Quinoa Bowl
Lunch: Lemony Farro and Sweet Potato Salad
Snack: Peanut Butter Banana Yogurt Bowls
Dinner: Cheese Spinach Stuffed Chicken Breasts
Dessert: Yogurt Pumpkin Parfait with Nuts

Week 2

Day 1:
Breakfast: Mango, Cucumber and Dates Smoothie
Lunch: Roasted Greens
Snack: Crispy Beet Chips
Dinner: BBQ Shrimp with Kale and Cheese Couscous
Dessert: Grilled Peaches with Yogurt Honey Dressing

Day 2:
Breakfast: Chocolate Almond Cookies
Lunch: Tofu and Tomato Scramble
Snack: Minty Tomato and Avocado Rolls
Dinner: White Fish and Potato Stew
Dessert: Homemade Chocolate Pancakes

Day 3:
Breakfast: Avocado Toast with Egg Salad
Lunch: Roasted Cauliflower
Snack: Cheese Pasta with Crab Rangoon Dip
Dinner: Spicy Flank Steak
Dessert: Chocolate Banana Smoothie Bowls

Day 4:
Breakfast: Muesli Scones
Lunch: Creamy Mushroom Pasta
Snack: Coconut and Nuts Trail Mix
Dinner: Lemony Pork Stew
Dessert: Blueberry and Dates Chia Pudding

Day 5:
Breakfast: Morning Tofu and Berries Smoothie
Lunch: Cumin Eggplant Tomato Stew
Snack: Herbed Potato Chips
Dinner: Spinach, Tofu, and Brown Rice Bowl
Dessert: Strawberry Chocolate Tofu Mousse

Day 6:
Breakfast: Chocolate Oats Cookie
Lunch: Avocado Bean Quesadilla
Snack: Beet-White Bean Hummus
Dinner: Pork with Tomatoes & Potatoes
Dessert: Coconut Mint Mousse

Day 7:
Breakfast: Bacon Egg Cups
Lunch: Lemony Cheese and Veggie Salad
Snack: Almonds and Cheese Stuffed Figs
Dinner: Garlicky Pork Stew
Dessert: Nutty Apple Porridge

Week 3

Day 1:
Breakfast: Spring Vegetables Frittata
Lunch: Cucumber and Quinoa Bowls
Snack: Almond-Walnuts Crackers
Dinner: Grilled Chicken with Cucumber-Radish Salad
Dessert: Mixed Berries with Coconut Cream

Day 2:
Breakfast: Tofu & Zucchini Muffins
Lunch: Chicken Pasta Soup
Snack: Delicious Hoisin Button Mushrooms
Dinner: Buttermilk Chicken with Almonds and Yogurt Dressing
Dessert: Classic Banana-Almond Cake

Day 3:
Breakfast: Strawberry and Kiwifruit Smoothie
Lunch: Lemony Black-Eyed Peas and Spinach Salad
Snack: Simple Boiled Unshelled Peanuts
Dinner: Lamb Chops with Mushrooms
Dessert: Nutty Protein Truffles

Day 4:
Breakfast: Sesame Seeds Bread
Lunch: Turkey, Spinach and Carrot Soup
Snack: Nutty Cranberry Oats
Dinner: Tomato Farro Spaghetti
Dessert: Strawberry-Applesauce Ice Cream

Day 5:
Breakfast: Blueberry Smoothie
Lunch: Beans and Grain Burgers
Snack: Spiced Nuts Mix
Dinner: Avocado-Tuna Stuffed Cucumber Roll
Dessert: Butter Apple Pie

Day 6:
Breakfast: Berries Quinoa Porridge
Lunch: Zucchini Noodles with Avocado Sauce
Snack: Crispy Flaxseed Crackers
Dinner: Mustard Chicken Nuggets
Dessert: Prosciutto Wrapped Plums

Day 7:
Breakfast: Mixed Berries Smoothie
Lunch: Salmon Watercress Pita Sandwich
Snack: Lemony Roasted Chickpeas
Dinner: Chicken Mushroom Meatloaf
Dessert: Chocolate Banana Bread

Week 4

Day 1:
Breakfast: Mushroom and Kale Quiche
Lunch: Cheese Prosciutto Corn Pizza
Snack: Peanut Butter Banana Yogurt Bowls
Dinner: Lemony Mustard Pork
Dessert: Yogurt Pumpkin Parfait with Nuts

Day 2:
Breakfast: Healthy Green Protein Smoothie
Lunch: Tomato Basil Pasta
Snack: Crispy Beet Chips
Dinner: Garlicky Balsamic Lamb Chops
Dessert: Grilled Peaches with Yogurt Honey Dressing

Day 3:
Breakfast: Veggie Frittata
Lunch: Spiced Beef Burgers
Snack: Minty Tomato and Avocado Rolls
Dinner: Cheese Spinach Stuffed Chicken Breasts
Dessert: Homemade Chocolate Pancakes

Day 4:
Breakfast: Carrot Cantaloupe Smoothie
Lunch: Tasty Steak and Potatoes
Snack: Cheese Pasta with Crab Rangoon Dip
Dinner: BBQ Shrimp with Kale and Cheese Couscous
Dessert: Blueberry and Dates Chia Pudding

Day 5:
Breakfast: Lime Avocado, Black Bean, and Quinoa Salad
Lunch: Mushroom-Avocado Tacos
Snack: Coconut and Nuts Trail Mix
Dinner: White Fish and Potato Stew
Dessert: Chocolate Banana Smoothie Bowls

Day 6:
Breakfast: Delicious Mushroom Omelet
Lunch: Lemony Salmon with Fennel Seeds
Snack: Herbed Potato Chips
Dinner: Pork with Tomatoes & Potatoes
Dessert: Strawberry Chocolate Tofu Mousse

Day 7:
Breakfast: Fruit and Green Tea Smoothie
Lunch: Millet with Eggplant Chickpea Stew
Snack: Almond-Walnuts Crackers
Dinner: Lamb Chops with Mushrooms
Dessert: Nutty Apple Porridge

Chapter 1 Breakfast and Smoothie Recipes

Chocolate Oats Cookie

Prep time: 8 minutes | Cook time: 15 minutes | Servings: 2

Ingredients:

2 medium ripe bananas, mashed

1 cup uncooked quick oats

¼ cup chocolate chips

Directions:

1. Preheat your oven to 350°F. Spray a non-stick cookie sheet with cooking spray. 2. In a bowl, mix the mashed bananas and oats. 3. Stir in the chocolate chips and spoon the equal mixture to the cookie sheet. 4. Bake for 15 minutes.

Per Serving: Calories 280; Fat 1.88g; Sodium 8mg; Carbs 69.77g; Fiber 8g; Sugar 50.88g; Protein 3.65g

Berries Quinoa Porridge

Prep time: 15 minutes | Cook time: 20 minutes | Servings: 4

Ingredients:

1 cup dry quinoa, rinsed

1½ cups unsweetened almond milk

1 teaspoon organic vanilla extract

1 teaspoon ground cinnamon

2 tablespoons maple syrup

4 tablespoons peanut butter

¼ cup fresh strawberries, hulled and chopped

¼ cup fresh blueberries

Directions:

1. Add the quinoa, vanilla extract, almond milk and cinnamon to a saucepan over medium heat and bring to a boil. 2. Reduce the heat, cover and simmer for 15 minutes or until the liquid is absorbed. 3. Remove the pan from heat and add the maple syrup and peanut butter. 4. Spread berries on top and Serve warm.

Per Serving: Calories 295; Fat 6.68g; Sodium 309mg; Carbs 51.26g; Fiber 4.4g; Sugar 20.85g; Protein 7.9g

Mixed Berries Smoothie

Prep time: 10 minutes | Cook time: 2 minutes | Servings: 5

Ingredients:

2½ cups whole strawberries, blueberries, raspberries, or chopped mango, divided

2½ cups sliced banana, divided

5 cups unsweetened vanilla almond milk or soymilk, divided

Directions:

1. Put ½ cup of strawberries (or another type of fruit) and ½ cup of banana into a resealable plastic sandwich bag. 2. Repeat this step four more times using the remaining fruit. 3. Keep the bags in the freezer until needed. 4. When ready to use, pour the contents of one bag and one cup of almond (or soy) milk into a blender and blend until smooth.

Per Serving: Calories 239; Fat 2.3g; Sodium 20mg; Carbs 52.43g; Fiber 5.1g; Sugar 39.24g; Protein 7.26g

Lime Avocado, Black Bean, and Quinoa Salad

Prep time: 20 minutes | Cook time: 0 minutes | Servings: 4

Ingredients:

2½ cups precooked quinoa

1 cup grape tomatoes

1 can black beans (10 ounces)

2 tablespoons extra-virgin olive oil

½ chopped avocado

¼ cup lime juice

1 cup cilantro leaves

½ teaspoon lime zest

½ teaspoon ground black pepper

1 clove garlic

¼ teaspoon salt

Directions:

1. In a large bowl, combine the quinoa, black beans, tomatoes and avocado. 2. In a food processor, blend the lime juice, olive oil, cilantro leaves, lime zest, salt, garlic clove, and black pepper. 3. Transfer this mixture to the quinoa bowl and toss well. 4. Refrigerate for 15 minutes.

Per Serving: Calories 493; Fat 13.25g; Sodium 216mg; Carbs 79.47g; Fiber 9.8g; Sugar 6.62g; Protein 16.13g

Sesame Bread

Prep time: 6 minutes | Cook time: 6 hours | Servings: 8

Ingredients:

4½ cups spelt flour	¼ cup agave
2 tsp sea salt	Grapeseed oil for brushing the bread
2 cups spring water	A dash of sesame seeds

Directions:

1. In a bowl, add the salt and spelt flour in a bowl, using a mixer's hook attachment and blend for 10 seconds. 2. Add the water and agave, mix for at least 10 minutes until a dough forms. 3. Brush the dough with grapeseed oil. Then place the dough in a bowl and let it rest for one hour. 4. Line the Instant Pot's base with a parchment paper. Sprinkle the dough with sesame seeds and place in the Instant Pot, close the lid. 5. Turn to the "Slow Cook" setting and cook for 6 hours.

Per Serving: Calories 178; Fat 2.37g; Sodium 587mg; Carbs 34.75g; Fiber 5.5g; Sugar 3.39g; Protein 7.34g

Chocolate Almond Cookies

Prep time: 15 minutes | Cook time: 10 minutes | Servings: 12

Ingredients:

1 cup gluten-free old-fashioned rolled oats	½ teaspoon baking powder
2 medium ripe bananas, mashed	¾ teaspoon pure vanilla extract
1 tablespoon unsalted almond butter	¼ teaspoon sea salt
2 tablespoons chia seeds	¼ cup dark chocolate chips

Directions:

1. Preheat your air fryer to 320°F. 2. Combine the oats, bananas, chia seeds, almond butter, vanilla, baking powder, and salt in a bowl. Gently add the chocolate chips, stir well. 3. Spoon the dough into the air fryer basket in a single layer, 1 inch apart. 4. Cook for about 10 minutes until golden brown. Serve cool.

Per Serving: Calories 55; Fat 1.02g; Sodium 72mg; Carbs 11.19g; Fiber 1.8g; Sugar 6.51g; Protein 0.98g

Mushroom and Kale Quiche

Prep time: 14 minutes | Cook time: 4 hours | Servings: 4

Ingredients:

1 cup garbanzos bean flour	2 cups mushrooms, sliced
¾ cup fresh coconut milk	1 cup kale, chopped
1 tbsp. sea salt	½ cup white onions, chopped
1 tbsp. oregano	½ cup yellow peppers, seeded and chopped
¼ teaspoon cayenne pepper	

Directions:

1. In a large bowl, combine the coconut milk, oregano, cayenne pepper, salt, garbanzo bean flour, knead to a smooth dough. 2. Add the remaining ingredients and mix well. Line Instant Pot with a parchment paper and pour the flour mixture inside, close the lid. 3. Turn to the "Slow Cook" setting and cook for 4 hours.

Per Serving: Calories 332; Fat 14.97g; Sodium 1810mg; Carbs 40.94g; Fiber 8.5g; Sugar 7.37g; Protein 12.26g

Bacon Egg Cups

Prep time: 10 minutes | Cook time: 17 minutes | Servings: 4

Ingredients:

6 sweet rolls	6 large cage free eggs
4 strips cooked bacon	Fresh cracked salt/pepper

Directions:

1. Preheat oven to 350°F. 2. Use a rolling pin to flip the rolls over. Try to make it as soft as possible without crumbling. 3. Place the rolls in a muffin tin sprinkled with non-stick spray. 4. Add a few pieces of chopped bacon to the muffin tin. 5. On the top of each muffin tin, crack an egg. 6. Sprinkle with salt and pepper to taste. 7. Transfer the muffin tin to the preheated oven and bake for 15-17 minutes until the egg whites are fully cooked. 8. When the cooking time is 5 minutes left, spread more pieces of bacon on top of the muffin.

Per Serving: Calories 204; Fat 4.5g; Sodium 723mg; Carbs 32.91g; Fiber 1.7g; Sugar 4.24g; Protein 7.21g

Spring Vegetables Frittata

Prep time: 10 minutes | Cook time: 20 minutes | Servings: 4

Ingredients:

2 tablespoons extra-virgin olive oil

½ small red onion, thinly sliced

1 jalapeño chile, thinly sliced (ribs and seeds removed for less heat, if desired)

1 zucchini, thinly sliced

¼ bunch asparagus (4 oz.), ends trimmed, tips cut into 2-inch pieces and stalks cut into ¼-inch pieces

Coarse salt

8 large eggs

Directions:

1. Preheat oven to 300°F. 2. Heat oil in an ovenproof skillet over medium heat. Add onion and jalapeño, saute for about 5 minutes until tender. Then add the zucchini and asparagus; cook for about 7 minutes more. Add salt to taste. 3. In a bowl, whisk the eggs and season with salt. Pour the egg mixture to the skillet with Vegetables; cook for 2 to 3 minutes until the edges just begin to set. 4. Place the skillet in the oven, broil for 2 to 3 minutes, until the middle part of the frittata is just set and the top is lightly golden and puffy. 5. Serve warm.

Per Serving: Calories 175; Fat 10.68g; Sodium 459mg; Carbs 5.63g; Fiber 1g; Sugar 3.84g; Protein 13.55g

Fruit and Green Tea Smoothie

Prep time: 4 minutes | Cook time: 2 minutes | Servings: 3

Ingredients:

2 cups frozen unsweetened mixed fruit, preferably peaches and pineapple

1 cup cold unsweetened green tea

1 tbsp honey

1 tablespoon lemon juice

Directions:

1. Mix the fruit, tea, honey, and lemon juice in a blender and blend until it becomes smooth and foamy. 2. Serve right away.

Per Serving: Calories 151; Fat 0.2g; Sodium 11mg; Carbs 41g; Fiber 2.3g; Sugar 38g; Protein 0.8g

Avocado Toast with Egg Salad

Prep time: 15 minutes | Cook time: 0 minutes | Servings: 2

Ingredients:

1 ½ tsp. reduced-Fat crumbled feta

3 cherry tomatoes, sliced

3 sliced Greek olives

1 slice whole-wheat bread

1 tbsp. hummus

¼ avocado, mashed

1 egg, hardboiled

Directions:

1. Toast the bread and spread the avocado and hummus on top. 2. Combine the cherry tomatoes, hard-boiled egg, olives, and feta in a bowl to make the salad. 3. Season with salt and pepper. 4. Serve the toast with salad

Per Serving: Calories 91; Fat 5.68g; Sodium 135mg; Carbs 8.5g; Fiber 2.6g; Sugar 1.6g; Protein 2.68g

Muesli Scones

Prep time: 10 minutes | Cook time: 12 minutes | Servings: 16

Ingredients:

½ tsp. celtic sea salt

¼ cup dried apricots, chopped

½ tsp. baking soda

2 cups almond flour, blanched

2 tbsp. honey

¼ cup dried cranberries

1 egg

¼ cup each of sesame seeds, sunflower seeds & pistachios, chopped

Directions:

1. Combine the flour, soda, salt, nuts, dried fruits, and seeds in a bowl, mix well. 2. In a separate bowl, whisk the egg and honey. Add dry ingredients to wet ingredients. 3. Knead into a dough using your hands. 4. Knead the dough ¾ inch thick and cut into 16 small pieces, making each piece into a square. 5. Preheat your oven to 350°F and line with a parchment baking sheet. 6. Put the dough squares in the oven and bake for 10-12 minutes.

Per Serving: Calories 75; Fat 5.18g; Sodium 135mg; Carbs 5.04g; Fiber 0.7g; Sugar 3.96g; Protein 2.98g

Chocolate Cherry Smoothie

Prep time: 4 minutes | Cook time: 00 minutes | Servings: 3

Ingredients:

½ cup oat milk	½ teaspoon vanilla extract
1 tbsp almond butter	1 cup frozen dark sweet cherries
1 teaspoon cocoa powder	1 tablespoon brown sugar, optional

Directions:

Blend all of the ingredients in a blender until fully combined.

Per Serving: Calories 107; Fat 5.3g; Sodium 68mg; Carbs 13.17g; Fiber 1g; Sugar 11.56g; Protein 2.21g

Veggie Frittata

Prep time: 10 minutes | Cook time: 25 minutes | Servings: 4

Ingredients:

¼ cup crème fraîche	2 cups cilantro leaves
6 large eggs	2 cups flat-leaf parsley leaves
2 tablespoons chives (chopped)	Pepper
4 tablespoons olive oil	½ cup dill fronds
6 scallions (one inch pieces)	Kosher salt

Directions:

1. In a bowl, mix together the crème fraîche and chives, refrigerate. 2. In a food processor, blend the scallions, cilantro, dill, parsley, and 2 tablespoons oil until finely chopped. Stir in eggs, ½ teaspoon salt and pepper. 3. Heat the remaining oil in a skillet over medium heat, about 2 minutes. Pour in the egg mixture and cook for 2 minutes until the edges begin to sizzle and set. 4. Preheat your oven to 350°F. Transfer the skillet to the oven. Bake for 18 to 20 minutes until the center is set. Let it rest for 5 minutes. 5. Garnish with chive crème fraîche.

Per Serving: Calories 238; Fat 21.15g; Sodium 232mg; Carbs 7.63g; Fiber 2.1g; Sugar 3.2g; Protein 5.91g

Delicious Mushroom Omelet

Prep time: 5 minutes | Cook time: 5 minutes | Servings: 1

Ingredients:

1 tablespoon olive oil

½ cup thinly sliced button mushrooms

Coarse salt and freshly ground pepper

¾ cup microgreens

3 large eggs

Directions:

1. In a nonstick skillet, heat 1½ teaspoons oil over medium-high heat. Add the mushrooms and cook for about 2 minutes until they begin to release liquid, add salt and pepper to taste. Stirring often, cook for additional 2 minutes. Then transfer the mushrooms to a bowl, add microgreens. 2. In a small bowl, whisk the eggs, add salt and pepper to taste. 3. In the skillet, heat remaining oil over medium heat. Then pour the egg mixture, cook until the edges are set, 1 to 2 minutes. 4. Put mushroom on one side of omelet, gently fold other side of omelet over the filling. 5. Serve warm.

Per Serving: Calories 497; Fat 31.91g; Sodium 912mg; Carbs 12.57g; Fiber 1.1g; Sugar 2.38g; Protein 38.65g

Chocolate-Blueberry Oatmeal

Prep time: 10 minutes | Cook time: 0 minutes | Servings: 2

Ingredients:

1 cup unsweetened almond milk

1 cup rolled oats

1 tbsp. cacao powder

8-10 drops liquid stevia

¼ cup fresh blueberries

1 tbsp. unsweetened dark mini chocolate chips

Directions:

1. Mix together all of the ingredients minus the blueberries and chocolate chips in a large bowl. 2. Cover, refridge Overnight in the refrigerator. 3. Top with blueberries and chocolate chips and serve.

Per Serving: Calories 233; Fat 6.4g; Sodium 73mg; Carbs 49.6g; Fiber 8g; Sugar 15.5g; Protein12.8 g

Sesame Seeds Bread

Prep time: 10 minutes | Cook time: 1 hour and 10 minutes | Servings: 8

Ingredients:

4 cups spelt flour

4 tablespoons sesame seeds

1 teaspoon baking soda

¼ teaspoon salt

10-12 drops liquid stevia

2 cups plus 2 tablespoons unsweetened almond milk

Directions:

1. Preheat the oven to 350°F. 2. Prepare a 9x5-inch loaf pan by lining it with greased parchment paper. Combine all the ingredients in a large bowl and mix until thoroughly incorporated. 3. Evenly transfer the mixture into the prepared loaf pan. Bake for about 1 hour and 10 minutes, or until a toothpick inserted into the center comes out clean. 4. Remove from the oven and place the loaf pan on a wire rack to cool for at least 10 minutes. 5. Gently invert the bread onto the rack to cool completely. 6. Using a sharp knife, slice the bread loaf into desired sizes and serve.

Per Serving: Calories 350; Fat 5.31g; Sodium 281mg; Carbs 67.45g; Fiber 10g; Sugar 11.49g; Protein 13.87g

Spinach-Grapefruit Pineapple Smoothie

Prep time: 8 minutes | Cook time: 2 minutes | Servings: 6

Ingredients:

1 cup plain coconut water

1 cup frozen diced pineapple

1 cup packed baby spinach

1 small grapefruit, peeled and segmented,

plus any juice squeezed from the membranes

½ teaspoon grated fresh ginger

1 cup ice

Directions:

1. Combine coconut water, ginger, and baby spinach in a blender along with pineapple, grapefruit, and ice. 2. Blend the mixture until it becomes smooth and frothy.

Per Serving: Calories 54; Fat 0.16g; Sodium 36mg; Carbs 13.27g; Fiber 1.3g; Sugar 11.87g; Protein 0.77g

Blueberry Smoothie

Prep time: 5 minutes | Cook time: 0 minutes| Servings: 3

Ingredients:

14 ounces canned unsweetened coconut milk

½ cup unsweetened almond milk

½ cup blueberries (fresh or frozen)

4 tablespoons pea protein powder

½ teaspoon vanilla extract

Directions:

1. Put blueberries, almond milk, pea protein powder, and vanilla in a powerful blender. 2. Slowly pour in coconut milk until the smoothie reaches the desired thickness. 3. Blend on high until all ingredients are fully mixed and the smoothie turns into a light purple shade. 4. Store the smoothie in a sealed container in the refrigerator for up to four days.

Per Serving: Calories 118; Fat 4.11g; Sodium 80mg; Carbs 13.18g; Fiber 0.6g; Sugar 11.29g; Protein 7.5g

Spiced Zucchini Strips

Prep time: 8 minutes plus 5 hours for marinating | Cook time: 6 minutes | Servings: 4

Ingredients:

3 zucchinis, sliced thinly lengthwise or into large strips

¼ cup date sugar

¼ cup spring water

1 tbsp. sea salt

1 tbsp. onion powder

½ teaspoon cayenne pepper powder

½ teaspoon ground ginger

1 tbsp. liquid smoke

Grapeseed oil for frying

Directions:

1. Mix all the ingredients except the oil in a bowl. Transfer to the refrigerator and marinate for at least two hours. 2. Turn your Instant Pot to Sauté setting, heat the oil on high heat until it begins to smoke slightly. 3. Place the marinated zucchini strips inside, cook for about 3 minutes on each side until crisp.

Per Serving: Calories 76; Fat 0.93g; Sodium 1766mg; Carbs 15.93g; Fiber 2.8g; Sugar 12.58g; Protein 3.31g

Carrot Cantaloupe Smoothie

Prep time: 15 minutes | Cook time: 2 minutes | Servings: 6

Ingredients:

4 cups frozen cubed cantaloupe (½-inch pieces)	Pinch of salt
¾ cup carrot juice	Melon balls, berries, nuts, or fresh basil for garnish

Directions:

1. To make the smoothie, put cantaloupe, carrot juice, and salt in a food processor or high-speed blender. 2. Pulse and blend the mixture for 1-2 minutes, stirring and scraping the sides occasionally to ensure it stays thick and smooth. 3. If desired, garnish the smoothie with extra melon, berries, almonds, or basil before serving.

Per Serving: Calories 289; Fat 1.5g; Sodium 994mg; Carbs 68.7g; Fiber 7g; Sugar 57g; Protein 7g

Morning Tofu and Berries Smoothie

Prep time: 15 minutes | Cook time: 2 minutes | Servings: 4

Ingredients:

1¼ cups orange juice, preferably calcium-fortified	blackberries, blueberries, or strawberries
1 banana	½ cup low-fat silken tofu, or low-fat plain yogurt
1¼ cups frozen berries, such as raspberries,	1 tbsp sugar, or Splenda Granular (optional)

Directions:

1. To make a smoothie, put orange juice, banana, strawberries, tofu (or yogurt), and sugar (or Splenda) in a blender. 2. Blend everything together until it becomes smooth and make sure to cover the blender. 3. Once done, serve the smoothie immediately.

Per Serving: Calories 166; Fat 1.3g; Sodium 18mg; Carbs 39g; Fiber 3.6g; Sugar 30.7g; Protein 2.6g

Strawberry and Kiwifruit Smoothie

Prep time: 5 minutes | Cook time: 2 minutes | Servings: 8

Ingredients:

4 cups sliced fresh strawberries	1 cup ice cubes
1 medium banana, sliced	1 kiwifruit, peeled and sliced, optional
1 (6-ounce) container vanilla low-fat yogurt	

Directions:

1. To make a smoothie, mix strawberries, banana, and yogurt in a blender until it becomes smooth. 2. Add ice cubes one at a time through the hole in the lid while the blender is running, and continue blending until smooth. 3. Pour the smoothie into eight small glasses and garnish with kiwifruit if desired. 4. Serve immediately.

Per Serving: Calories 61; Fat 0.7g; Sodium 17mg; Carbs 13g; Fiber 2.4g; Sugar 8.5g; Protein 2g

Healthy Green Protein Smoothie

Prep time: 5 minutes | Cook time: 0 minutes Servings: 1

Ingredients:

4 cubes ice	⅛ cup fresh mint leaves
½ cup spinach	1 scoop vanilla whey protein powder
½ cup soy milk	1 tbsp almonds

Directions:

Combine almonds, spinach, protein powder, soy milk, and icing in a blender cup and blend until the mixture becomes smooth.

Per Serving: Calories 267; Fat 13.58g; Sodium 142mg; Carbs 19.72g; Fiber 2.8g; Sugar 11.51g; Protein 18.14g

Apple Spinach-Curry Crepes

Prep time: 10 minutes | Cook time: 20 minutes | Servings:2

Ingredients:

2 large eggs

⅓ cup finely chopped fresh cilantro

¼ teaspoon black pepper

2½ cups 1% milk

1 cup plus 2 tablespoons all-purpose flour

3 tablespoons safflower oil

¾ teaspoon kosher salt

1 small chopped yellow onion

1 can rinsed and drained chickpeas

1 diced apple

¼ cup golden raisins

2 tablespoons madras curry powder

10 ounces fresh spinach

Lemon wedges

Directions:

1. Blend the eggs, cilantro, 1 cup flour, 2 tbsp. oil, pepper, 1 cup milk, and ¼ tsp. salt in a blender. 2. Grease a 10-inch skillet with non-stick cooking spray. 3. Place ⅓ cup batter in the pan and cook over medium heat around 1 minute. Flip and cook for 30 seconds. Repeat with the remaining batter. 4. Heat the remaining oil in a pan over medium heat. Sauté the onion for about 5 minutes until soft. 5. Add the chickpeas, apple, curry powder, and raisins, sauté for 3 minutes. 6. Then stir in the remaining flour and cook for additional 30 seconds. 7. Add the remaining milk and cook for 2 minutes or until thick. 8. Finally add the spinach and the remaining ½ teaspoon salt and cook for 2 minutes until wilted. 9. Divide evenly among the crepes, fold in half, and spread lemon slices on top. Serve.

Per Serving: Calories 1007; Fat 40.44g; Sodium 1403mg; Carbs 134.82g; Fiber 20g; Sugar 45.31g; Protein 34.15g

Nutty Chicken Quinoa Bowl

Prep time: 15 minutes | Cook time: 18 minutes | Servings: 4

Ingredients:

1-pound chicken breasts (boneless, skinless)	1 tsp. paprika
¼ tsp. salt	2 tbsps. finely chopped fresh parsley
1 (7 oz.). jar roasted red peppers	2 cups cooked quinoa
¼ tsp. ground pepper	¼ teaspoon crushed red pepper
½ tsp. ground cumin	¼ cup chopped pitted Kalamata olives
¼ cup slivered almonds	1 cup diced cucumber
1 small crushed clove garlic	¼ cup finely chopped red onion
4 tbsps. extra-virgin olive oil	¼ cup crumbled feta cheese

Directions:

1. Place a rack in the upper third of the oven and preheat the oven to high temperature. Wrap a framed baking sheet with aluminum foil. 2. Spread the chicken seasoned with pepper and salt in a single layer on a baking sheet. Bake for 14 to 18 minutes, turning once. Then cut the chicken into slices or strips. 3. In the meantime, Puree the almonds, peppers, cumin, 2 tbsps oil, paprika, garlic, and cracked red pepper in a food processor until smooth. 4. Mix the quinoa, olives, red onion, and remaining oil in a bowl. 5. Divide the quinoa mixture evenly over four bowls. Pour in equal amounts of chicken, cucumber, and red pepper sauce. 6. Serve with parsley and feta on top.

Per Serving: Calories 493; Fat 29.22g; Sodium 490mg; Carbs 27.37g; Fiber 5g; Sugar 4.23g; Protein 30.9g

Tofu & Zucchini Muffins

Prep time: 15 minutes | Cook time: 40 minutes | Servings: 6

Ingredients:

12 ounces extra-firm silken tofu, drained and pressed

¾ cup unsweetened soy milk

2 tablespoons canola oil

1 tablespoon apple cider vinegar

1 cup whole-wheat pastry flour

½ cup chickpea flour

1 teaspoon baking powder

½ teaspoon baking soda

1 teaspoon smoked paprika

1 teaspoon onion powder

1 teaspoon salt

½ cup zucchini, chopped

¼ cup fresh chives, minced

Directions:

1. Preheat the oven to 400ºF. 2. To make muffins, first line a 12-cup muffin tin with paper liners. 3. In a bowl, mash tofu with a fork until it becomes smooth. Add almond milk, oil, and vinegar to the tofu and mix until it becomes slightly smooth. 4. In a separate bowl, mix together the flours, baking soda, baking powder, spices, and salt. 5. Transfer the mixture evenly into the prepared muffin cups. Bake the muffins for about 35-40 minutes or until a toothpick inserted in the center comes out clean. 6. Once the muffins are cooked, remove the muffin tin from the oven and place it on a wire rack to cool for around 10 minutes. 7. Then, carefully invert the muffins onto a platter and serve them warm.

Per Serving: Calories 209; Fat 9.66g; Sodium 521mg; Carbs 22.63g; Fiber 3.5g; Sugar 2.89g; Protein 10.6g

Mango, Cucumber and Dates Smoothie

Prep time: 5 minutes | Cook time: 0 minutes Servings: 2

Ingredients:

½ cup crushed ice or 3-4 ice cubes	1 small cucumber, peeled and chopped
1 cup coconut milk	1-2 dates, pitted
1 mango, peeled and diced	1 tbsp chia seeds

Directions:

Blend all the ingredients in a high-speed blender until they are smooth. Then, serve and enjoy!

Per Serving: Calories 236; Fat 7.08g; Sodium 57mg; Carbs 39.88g; Fiber 6.2g; Sugar 33.59g; Protein 7.06g

Chapter 2 Vegan and Vegetarian Recipes

Herbed Veggie Stew

Prep time: 10 minutes | Cook time: 15 minutes | Servings: 8

Ingredients:

¼ cup extra-virgin olive oil

3 leeks, thinly sliced

1 cup chopped red potatoes

1 cup peeled and sliced parsnips

1 cup peeled and chopped turnip

1 cup sliced celery

1 cup sliced carrots

4 cups garbanzo beans, drained

4 cups low-sodium vegetable broth

2 cups vegan stout beer (such as Samuel Smith's)

½ cup chopped fresh parsley

¼ teaspoon dried rosemary

¼ teaspoon dried thyme

¼ teaspoon dried marjoram

¼ cup water (optional)

Salt and ground black pepper to taste

Directions:

1. Put the appropriate pot on the stove and set the heat to medium-high. 2. Next, add olive oil and heat it up before adding leeks. Cook the leeks for 3 to 5 minutes until they become translucent. 3. Then, add potatoes, parsnips, celery, turnips, and carrots to the pot. Cook and stir for 4 minutes until they are slightly soft and coated in oil. 4. Optional ingredients such as parsley, vegetable broth, garbanzo beans, and beer can be added to the mix. 5. Allow the stew to boil. Keep cooking the mixture for an hour or two until the vegetables become tender and the stew has thickened. 6. Lastly, add the herbs and season with salt and pepper to taste. 7. Add a splash of water if necessary.

Per Serving: Calories 168; Fat 2.3g; Sodium 526mg; Carbs 33g; Fiber 7g; Sugar 10g; Protein 5.9g

Mayo Coleslaw

Prep time: 10 minutes plus 2 hours for chilling | Cook time: 15 minutes | Servings: 2

Ingredients:

1 (16 ounces) bag coleslaw mix

⅔ cup vegan mayonnaise

½ cup granular sucralose sweetener

3 tbsps olive oil

1 tbsp. white vinegar

1 tbsp. poppy seeds

¼ teaspoon salt

Directions:

1. Put the coleslaw mix into a suitable mixing bowl and mix well. 2. In a mixing bowl, mix together vegan mayonnaise, sweetener, vinegar, poppy seeds, olive oil, and salt. 3. Slowly mix the coleslaw into the dressing until fully coated. 4. Refrigerate the coleslaw for a minimum of two hours before serving. 5. Serve chilled.

Per Serving: Calories 521; Fat 48g; Sodium 1013mg; Carbs 16g; Fiber 6g; Sugar 3g; Protein 9g

Tangy Mushroom Stroganoff

Prep time: 10 minutes | Cook time: 15 minutes | Servings: 1

Ingredients:

8 ounces oyster mushrooms

1 tbsp. oil, or to taste

1 small onion, diced

1 tbsp. all-purpose flour

1 cup almond milk

1 tbsp. lemon juice

Salt and ground black pepper to taste

Directions:

1. With a fork, shred the mushrooms. Put a skillet on the stove and set the heat to medium-high. 2. Once the oil is heated, add the mushrooms and onion and cook for 2 to 3 minutes, or until the vegetables are tender. 3. While stirring, add the flour and let it simmer for a bit. 4. In a bowl, mix almond milk and lemon juice, add to the skillet. Cook for 7 to 8 minutes. 5. Add salt and pepper to taste.

Per Serving: Calories 989; Fat 19g; Sodium 206mg; Carbs 211g; Fiber 29g; Sugar 31.7g; Protein 26g

Avocado Bean Quesadilla

Prep time: 10 minutes | Cook time: 15 minutes | Servings: 4

Ingredients:

1 avocado

4 tortillas

¼ cup vegetable broth

¼ teaspoon cumin

¼ teaspoon chili powder

¼ teaspoon garlic powder

¼ teaspoon onion powder

1 adobo chipotle pepper

15 oz. rinsed & drained pinto beans

Directions:

1. Combine all the ingredients except the tortillas in a food processor or blender and blend until smooth. 2. If necessary, add additional broth to achieve the desired consistency. 3. Spread the mixture along one side of a tortilla, fold the tortilla, and place it on a non-stick pan. Cook both sides until golden brown. 4. Remove from heat, cut into pieces, and serve.

Per Serving: Calories 249; Fat 10.69g; Sodium 380mg; Carbs 34.59g; Fiber 6.8g; Sugar 3.46g; Protein 6.24g

Roasted Greens

Prep time: 10 minutes | Cook time: 17 minutes | Servings: 2

Ingredients:

6 to 8 oz. hearty greens, such as kale, chard, mustard, collards or spinach

¼ cup olive oil (not extra-virgin)

¼ teaspoon kosher salt

Directions:

1. Preheat the oven to 300°F. Line two half sheet pans with parchment paper. Wash and completely dry the greens. Tear the larger leaves into strips that are 1 to 2 inches in size. 2. Arrange the greens in a single layer on the half sheet pans, lightly spray them with olive oil and sprinkle with salt. 3. Bake the greens for 15 to 20 minutes, until they are dry and have darkened slightly. Immediately remove them from the pan onto the parchment and transfer them to the serving plate. 4. Repeat with the remaining greens. Serve.

Per Serving: Calories 287; Fat 27.92g; Sodium 329mg; Carbs 8.68g; Fiber 3.6g; Sugar 2.24g; Protein 4.25g

Roasted Cauliflower

Prep time: 5 minutes | Cook time: 25 minutes | Servings: 2

Ingredients:

½ head cauliflower	Salt
1 tablespoon extra-virgin olive oil	1 teaspoon red-pepper flakes

Directions:

1. Preheat the oven to 425°F. Spread ½ head of cauliflower, cut into florets, onto a rimmed baking sheet. 2. Drizzle 1 tablespoon of extra-virgin olive oil over the cauliflower and season with coarse salt. 3. Toss the cauliflower to combine, then spread it out in a single layer. Roast the cauliflower, tossing it halfway through cooking, until it is golden brown and just tender, which should take approximately 25 minutes. 4. Sprinkle with red pepper flakes. Serve.

Per Serving: Calories 99; Fat 7.32g; Sodium 393mg; Carbs 7.82g; Fiber 3.2g; Sugar 2.9g; Protein 2.93g

Tofu and Tomato Scramble

Prep time: 15 minutes | Cook time: 15 minutes | Servings: 2

Ingredients:

½ tablespoon olive oil	1½ cups firm tofu, pressed, drained and crumbled
1 small onion, chopped finely	
1 small red bell pepper, seeded and chopped finely	Pinch of cayenne pepper
	Pinch of ground turmeric
1 cup cherry tomatoes, chopped finely	Salt, as required

Directions:

1. Heat oil in a skillet over medium heat and sauté onion and bell pepper for approximately 4-5 minutes. 2. Add tomatoes and cook for around 1-2 minutes. Add tofu, cayenne pepper, turmeric, and salt, and cook for roughly 6-8 minutes, stirring often. 3. Serve while hot.

Per Serving: Calories 238; Fat 11.74g; Sodium 616mg; Carbs 20.85g; Fiber 4.9g; Sugar 13.57g; Protein 17.38g

Tasty Quinoa and Roasted Vegetables

Prep time: 10 minutes | Cook time: 20 minutes | Servings: 2

Ingredients:

½ butternut squash, peeled and diced

20 Brussels sprouts, trimmed and halved

¼ cup melted coconut oil or extra-virgin olive oil

Coarse salt and freshly ground pepper

1 teaspoon smoked paprika (pimenton)

¾ cup plus 2 tablespoons water

½ cup quinoa, rinsed and drained

1 garlic clove

2 tablespoons tahini

3 tablespoons apple cider vinegar

¼ cup snipped fresh chives

¼ cup chopped fresh flat-leaf parsley leaves

¼ cup chopped fresh cilantro leaves

2½ cups baby spinach

Directions:

1. Preheat the oven to 425°F. On a baking sheet, mix the squash and Brussels sprouts with 2 tablespoons of olive oil, season with salt and paprika. 2. Roast the vegetables, stirring halfway through, until they are golden and tender, about 25 to 30 minutes. 3. In the meantime, in a medium saucepan, bring the quinoa, ¾ cup of water, and a pinch of salt to a boil. Turn down the heat, cover, and simmer until the liquid is absorbed and the quinoa is tender but chewy, around 15 minutes. Transfer to a bowl and fluff with a fork. 4. In a food processor, pulse garlic, tahini, remaining 2 tablespoons of oil, vinegar, remaining 2 tablespoons of water, parsley, chives, and cilantro until smooth. Season with salt and pepper. 5. In a mixing bowl, combine roasted vegetables and quinoa with 2 tablespoons of sauce. 6. For each serving, add spinach and season with salt and pepper.

Per Serving: Calories 539; Fat 30.9g; Sodium 412mg; Carbs 57.05g; Fiber 13.6g; Sugar 6.96g; Protein 15.11g

Lemony Farro and Sweet Potato Salad

Prep time: 10 minutes | Cook time: 40 minutes | Servings: 4

Ingredients:

2 pounds sweet potatoes (about 4), scrubbed and cut into 1-inch pieces

3 garlic cloves (do not peel)

¼ cup plus 1 tablespoon extra-virgin olive oil

Coarse salt and freshly ground pepper

1 cup farro

Grated zest and juice of 1 lemon (about 3 tablespoons)

½ cup fresh dill, chopped

½ cup spicy sprouts, such as radish or arugula, plus more for garnish

Directions:

1. Preheat the oven to 425°F. Drizzle 3 tablespoons of oil over sweet potatoes and garlic on two rimmed baking sheets. 2. Season with salt and pepper, toss to combine, then spread in a single layer. 3. Roast the sweet potatoes, flipping once, until they are tender and caramelized, which takes about 30 minutes. 4. In the meantime, place farro in a medium saucepan and cover it with 4 inches of water. 5. Bring it to a boil, then reduce the heat and let it simmer until tender for around 30 to 35 minutes. 6. Drain the farro and immediately toss it with the remaining 2 tablespoons of oil in a bowl. Season with salt and let it cool down slightly. 7. Remove garlic cloves from their skins and use a mortar and pestle to mash them with lemon zest and juice. 8. Add the mixture to farro, then add the sweet potatoes, sprouts and dill, mix well. 9. Season with salt and pepper. Garnish with additional sprouts before serving.

Per Serving: Calories 405; Fat 18.65g; Sodium 212mg; Carbs 53.21g; Fiber 15.4g; Sugar 1.17g; Protein 12.45g

Creamy Mushroom Pasta

Prep time: 10 minutes | Cook time: 20 minutes | Servings: 4

Ingredients:

1 small finely diced yellow onion	¾ cup vegan sour cream
3 minced garlic cloves	1¼ cups low-sodium vegetable stock
4 tablespoons extra-virgin olive oil	2 tablespoons chopped parsley
2 tablespoons whole-wheat flour	Sea salt as needed
2 lbs. trimmed & sliced cremini mushrooms	Black pepper as needed
¾ cup dry white wine	16 oz. whole-wheat pasta

Directions:

1. As per the package instructions, cook the noodles until they reach the dente stage. Once done, drain the noodles and reserve half a cup of pasta water. 2. Next, melt some butter in a medium-sized pot over medium-high heat. Add the onion and sauté until it turns golden brown, which should take around 5 minutes. Add the garlic and mushrooms, and continue cooking for an additional 5 minutes until the mushrooms become tender. 3. Stir in the flour and make sure there are no white streaks in the mixture. Cook for a minute before adding the wine and vegetable stock. Keep the flame at medium and cook for 5 minutes or until the sauce thickens. 4. Add in the sour cream and season with salt and pepper as required. Combine the pasta with the mushroom sauce and mix well. 5. If the sauce is too thick, you can use the reserved pasta water to make it more liquid. 6. Serve the dish in bowls with the creamy sauce on top.

Per Serving: Calories 730; Fat 28.55g; Sodium 828mg; Carbs 102.89g; Fiber 18.3g; Sugar 8.64g; Protein 26.94g

Cumin Eggplant Tomato Stew

Prep time: 5 minutes | Cook time: 10 minutes | Servings: 4

Ingredients:

1 cup diced onions	⅛ teaspoon ground cayenne pepper
3½ cups cubed eggplants	1 teaspoon ground cumin
1 cup tomato sauce	1 teaspoon sea salt
2 cups diced tomatoes	½ cup water

Directions:

1. Switch on the instant pot and add in all the ingredients. Give it a stir to blend and then cover the pot. 2. Press the manual button and cook for 5 minutes on high until it's fully cooked. 3. After it's done, release the steam, cautiously open the pot, and mix it up. 4. Serve the hot stew and add salt to taste if necessary.

Per Serving: Calories 116; Fat 0.63g; Sodium 1502mg; Carbs 23.68g; Fiber 7.6g; Sugar 12.99g; Protein 3.5g

Baked Potatoes and Sweet Lentils

Prep time: 10 minutes | Cook time: 15 minutes | Servings: 4

Ingredients:

4 sliced large baked potatoes	1 tsp. liquid smoke
1 cup dry brown lentils	1 cup water
1 tsp. molasses	½ cup organic ketchup
1 chopped small onion	

Directions:

1. Add onion, water, and lentils to the pot. Secure the lid and cook on high pressure for 10 minutes. 2. Allow the pressure to release naturally. Then add the ketchup, molasses, and liquid smoke to the lentils. Sauté for 5 minutes. 3. Serve over the baked potatoes.

Per Serving: Calories 373; Fat 0.68g; Sodium 370mg; Carbs 82.38g; Fiber 12.1g; Sugar 11.84g; Protein 12.44g

Herbed Spinach Lasagna

Prep time: 15 minutes | Cook time: 50 minutes | Servings: 8

Ingredients:

2 tbsps olive oil

1½ cup chopped onion

3 tbsps minced garlic

4 (14.5 ounces) cans stewed tomatoes

⅓ cup tomato paste

½ cup chopped fresh basil

½ cup chopped parsley

1 teaspoon salt

1 teaspoon ground black pepper

1 (16 ounces) package lasagna noodles

2 pounds firm tofu

2 tbsps minced garlic

¼ cup chopped fresh basil

¼ cup chopped parsley

½ teaspoon salt

Ground black pepper to taste

3 (10 ounces) packages frozen chopped spinach, thawed and drained

Directions:

To make the tomato sauce:

1. To prepare the sauce, you will need a large and sturdy saucepan. 2. Heat the olive oil over medium heat and add the onions, sautéing them for about 5 minutes until they become soft. 3. Next, add the garlic and cook for an additional 5 minutes. 4. In a separate saucepan, combine the tomatoes, tomato paste, basil, and parsley. Give the mixture a good stir, then lower the heat and cover the saucepan for an hour to let the flavors meld. 5. In the meantime, bring a large saucepan of salted water to a boil for the lasagna noodles. Boil the noodles for 9 minutes, then drain and rinse them thoroughly. 6. Preheat the oven to 400°F. Combine all of the blocks of tofu in a large mixing bowl. 7. In a separate mixing dish, mix together the parsley, basil, and garlic. Add salt and pepper to the tofu and use your fingers to squeeze and mix everything together until thoroughly combined.

To make the lasagna:

1. Start by spreading 1 cup of tomato sauce on the bottom of a casserole pan measuring 9x13 inches. 2. Place a layer of lasagna noodles, followed by ⅓ of the tofu mixture. Distribute the spinach evenly over the tofu. 3. Add another layer of noodles on top of the tofu, followed by 1 and a half cups of tomato sauce. 4. Then, add another ⅓ of the tofu mixture on top of the noodles, followed by 1½ cups of tomato sauce. 5. Add one final layer of noodles on top of the tomato sauce to finish the dish. 6. To complete, pour the remaining tomato sauce over the noodles and evenly distribute the remaining ⅓ of the tofu on top. 7. Cover the lasagna with foil and bake in the oven for 30 minutes. 8. Serve immediately and savor the delicious flavors.

Per Serving: Calories 377; Fat 17.7g; Sodium 1043mg; Carbs 34g; Fiber 12.7g; Sugar 10.7g; Protein 30g

Parsley Radish and Tomato Salad

Prep time: 8 minutes | Cook time: 0 minutes | Servings: 3-4

Ingredients:

1 medium head romaine lettuce, torn	½ cup flat-leaf parsley, chopped
3 small tomatoes, diced	⅓ cup olive oil or avocado oil
1 medium cucumber, sliced	3 tbsps lemon juice
1 small green bell pepper, sliced	1 garlic clove, minced
1 small onion, cut into rings	Salt & pepper
6 radishes, thinly sliced	1 teaspoon fresh mint, minced

Directions:

1. Combine the lettuce, tomatoes, onion, cucumber, pepper, radishes, and parsley in a salad bowl. 2. In a separate bowl, mix together the olive oil, lemon juice, garlic, mint, salt, and pepper. 3. Drizzle the mixture over the salad and toss until well-coated.

Per Serving: Calories 110; Fat 6.8g; Sodium 178mg; Carbs 11.6g; Fiber 4.5g; Sugar 5.6g; Protein 3g

Avocado, Olives and Tomato Salad

Prep time: 5 minutes | Cook time: 0 minutes | Servings: 4

Ingredients:

2 tbsp. olive oil	1 cup tomatoes, cubed
2 avocados, cut into wedges	1 tbsp. ginger, grated
1 cup Kalamata olives, pitted and halved	Pinch black pepper
1 tbsp. balsamic vinegar	2 cups baby arugula

Directions:

Mix together the Kalamata olives with the avocados and other ingredients in a bowl, toss well, and serve as a side dish.

Per Serving: Calories 247; Fat 22.74g; Sodium 122mg; Carbs 12.27g; Fiber 7.8g; Sugar 2.72g; Protein 2.84g

Lemony Tuna and Beans Salad

Prep time: 8 minutes | Cook time: 0 minutes | Servings: 1

Ingredients:

1 can tuna in water, drained

⅓ cup four bean mix (or just white or red beans), drained, rinsed

1 tomato, deseeded, chopped

1 large celery stick, trimmed, finely chopped

½ small onion, halved, thinly sliced

½ cup flat-leaf parsley leaves, chopped

½ lemon, rind finely grated, juiced

1 garlic clove, crushed

1 tbsp. extra-virgin olive oil

Directions:

In a mixing bowl, mix together all of the ingredients, then plate.

Per Serving: Calories 399; Fat 17g; Sodium 661mg; Carbs 26g; Fiber 7.5g; Sugar 5.7g; Protein 39g

Cucumber and Yogurt Salad

Prep time: 4 minutes | Cook time: 0 minutes | Servings: 2-3

Ingredients:

2-3 cucumbers, sliced

2 tsp salt

3 tbsps lemon juice

¼ teaspoon paprika

¼ teaspoon white pepper

½ clove garlic, minced

4 fresh green onions, diced

1 cup thick Greek yogurt

¼ teaspoon paprika

Directions:

1. Thinly slice the cucumbers and sprinkle them with salt. 2. Allow yourself an hour to prepare. Prepare a mixture of white pepper, garlic, paprika, lemon juice, and water and set it aside. 3. Squeeze each slice of cucumber dry and transfer it to a bowl, discarding any excess liquid. 4. In a separate mixing bowl, combine the yogurt, green onions, and lemon juice. Add the cucumber slices to the bowl and mix everything together. Sprinkle paprika or dill on top. 5. Cover the bowl and refrigerate for a few hours.

Per Serving: Calories 212; Fat 1g; Sodium 1617mg; Carbs 41g; Fiber 5.4g; Sugar 27g; Protein 12g

Cucumber-Watercress Salad

Prep time: 5 minutes | Cook time: 5 minutes | Servings: 2

Ingredients:

2 cups torn watercress	2 tbsps olive oil
½ cucumber, sliced	pure sea salt, to taste
1 tbsp. key lime juice	cayenne powder, to taste

Directions:

1. Add olive oil and key lime juice to a salad bowl, and mix them thoroughly. 2. Next, slice a cucumber and add all the slices to the bowl. 3. Tear up some watercress and add it to the bowl. 4. Season with salt and cayenne pepper to your liking, and finish off with a sprinkle of pure sea salt on top. 5. Your detox salad is now ready to be enjoyed!

Per Serving: Calories 125; Fat 13.5g; Sodium 14mg; Carbs 1g; Fiber 0.2g; Sugar 0.2g; Protein 0.8g

Lemony Cheese and Veggie Salad

Prep time: 10 minutes | Cook time: 0 minutes | Servings: 4

Ingredients:

1 head iceberg lettuce	4 ounces sliced radishes
1 head romaine lettuce	4 ounces low-fat feta or goat cheese
1 pound plump tomatoes	2 ounces anchovies (optional)
6 ounces Greek or black olives, sliced	

Dressing:

3 ounces olive oil or avocado oil	1 teaspoon black pepper
3 ounces fresh lemon juice	1 teaspoon salt
1 teaspoon dried oregano	4 cloves garlic, minced

Directions:

1. It is necessary to wash the lettuce before cutting it into small pieces. It is suggested to cut the tomatoes into quarters. 2. In a large bowl, mix together the olives, tomatoes, lettuce, and radishes. 3. Combine the dressing with the vegetables. Fill a small serving bowl halfway with the mixture. 4. Add crumbled feta or goat cheese on top, and optionally, anchovy fillets.

Per Serving: Calories 407; Fat 32g; Sodium 1607mg; Carbs 23g; Fiber 8.8g; Sugar 8g; Protein 12g

Cucumber and Quinoa Bowls

Prep time: 10 minutes | Cook time: 0 minutes | Servings: 2

Ingredients:

1 cup cooked quinoa mixed

1 tbsp. sesame seeds

½ cup chopped tomato and green pepper

1 cup chopped cucumber

½ cup chopped cilantro

Dressing:

1 tbsp. olive oil or cumin oil

1 tbsp. fresh lemon juice

1 pinch black pepper

1 pinch sea salt

Directions:

Combine all the ingredients in a large mixing bowl.

Per Serving: Calories 237; Fat 11.6g; Sodium 741mg; Carbs 29g; Fiber 5g; Sugar 6.6g; Protein 6g

Lemony Black-Eyed Peas and Spinach Salad

Prep time: 15 minutes | Cook time: 6 minutes | Servings: 2

Ingredients:

1 tablespoon olive oil

3 cups purple cabbage, chopped

5 cups baby spinach

1 cup shredded carrots

1 can black-eyed peas, drained

Juice of ½ lemon

Pinch salt

1 teaspoon freshly ground black pepper

Directions:

1. Heat oil in a medium pan and sauté cabbage over medium heat for 1 to 2 minutes. 2. Add spinach, cover, and cook over medium heat for 3 to 4 minutes until wilted. 3. Transfer to a large bowl. Add carrots, black-eyed peas, and a splash of lemon juice. 4. Season with salt and pepper. Toss and serve.

Per Serving: Calories 305; Fat 3.88g; Sodium 330mg; Carbs 54.45g; Fiber 18.5g; Sugar 27.18g; Protein 18.44g

Tomato-Bean Soup

Prep time: 15 minutes | Cook time: 1 hour 10 minutes | Servings: 6-8

Ingredients:

10 chopped plum tomatoes	1 teaspoon sweet basil
1 chopped tomatillo	1 teaspoon oregano
3 cups cooked garbanzo beans	½ teaspoon achiote
½ cup chopped red bell pepper	2 tsp pure sea salt
½ cup minced onions	2 tsp grapeseed oil
½ cup chopped green bell pepper	Spring water, to cook
2 tsp onion powder	Sausage, for serving
1 teaspoon cayenne powder	

Directions:

1. Combine bell pepper, grapeseed oil, onions, and tomatillo in a large pot. 2. Cook the vegetables over medium heat for 4 to 5 minutes. 3. Add Garbanzo beans, spices, tomatoes, and spring water to the pot. Stir and bring the mixture to a boil. 4. Reduce the heat and simmer the tomato-bean mixture for about an hour, stirring occasionally. 5. If desired, add sliced sausage links a few minutes before the soup is done cooking. 6. Serve the soup and enjoy!

Per Serving: Calories 87; Fat 1.6g; Sodium 217mg; Carbs 18.8g; Fiber 2.4g; Sugar 14.5g; Protein 1.4g

Turkey, Spinach and Carrot Soup

Prep time: 20 minutes | Cook time: 20 minutes | Servings: 6

Ingredients:

5 carrots, chopped	½ tsp. pepper
2 cups baby spinach	1 tbsp. canola oil
1 onion, chopped	⅔ cup quick-cooking barley
2 cups cooked turkey breast, cubed	6 cups chicken broth, low-sodium

Directions:

1. Sauté the onions and carrots in hot oil for 4 to 5 minutes. Add the remaining ingredients.
2. Allow it to come to a boil, then reduce the heat and let it simmer for 10 to 15 minutes.

Per Serving: Calories 136; Fat 5.51g; Sodium 230mg; Carbs 12.13g; Fiber 2.7g; Sugar 3.28g; Protein 9.78g

Chickpea and Spinach Soup

Prep time: 10 minutes | Cook time: 22 minutes | Servings: 6

Ingredients:

2 tbsp. minced garlic

1 tsp. cumin

15 oz. canned tomatoes, diced, with liquid

¼ tsp. pepper

14.5 oz. canned vegetable broth: low-

sodium

1 small onion (chopped)

16 oz. canned chickpeas, with liquid

4 cups fresh spinach, packed

Directions:

1. Heat some oil over medium heat in a medium-sized pot. Sauté garlic and onion for 5 minutes. 2. Add all the other ingredients except for spinach, stir, and bring to a boil. 3. Reduce the heat, add spinach, cook for 10 to 15 minutes. 4. Serve.

Per Serving: Calories 156; Fat 2.02g; Sodium 547mg; Carbs 30.53g; Fiber 7.3g; Sugar 12.11g; Protein 8.05g

Spinach, Endives and Walnuts Salad

Prep time: 5 minutes | Cook time: 0 minutes | Servings: 4

Ingredients:

2 endives, roughly shredded

1 tbsp. dill, chopped

¼ cup lemon juice

¼ cup olive oil

2 cups baby spinach

2 tomatoes, cubed

1 cucumber, sliced

½ cups walnuts, chopped

Directions:

In a bowl, mix together the spinach, endives and remaining ingredients, toss well and serve as a side dish.

Per Serving: Calories 245; Fat 23.59g; Sodium 18mg; Carbs 8.16g; Fiber 2.9g; Sugar 3.15g; Protein 3.87g

Chickpea and Cucumber Salad

Prep time: 10 minutes | Cook time: 10 minutes | Servings: 4

Ingredients:

1 (15 oz.) can chickpeas, drained and rinsed

1 tablespoon olive oil

1 teaspoon cumin

1 teaspoon paprika

¼ teaspoon cilantro

¼ teaspoon cinnamon

½ teaspoon salt

Hummus Dressing:

¼ cup hummus

2 tablespoons tahini

Juice from half a lemon

¼ teaspoon ground black pepper

2 romaine lettuce hearts, cut into wedges

½ medium cucumber, thinly sliced into half moons

½ small red onion, thinly sliced into half moons

2 roasted red peppers, thinly sliced

¼ cup feta cheese, crumbled

½ teaspoon salt

3 tablespoons olive oil

Directions:

1. First, heat the oven to 400°F. 2. Then, dry the chickpeas completely by placing them on a paper or kitchen towel. 3. In a medium-sized bowl, mix together the chickpeas, olive oil, cumin, paprika, cilantro, cinnamon, salt, and pepper. 4. Once combined, spread the chickpea mixture on a large baking sheet lined with parchment paper, ensuring that they are in a single layer. 5. Bake for 25 minutes, shaking the pan halfway through to ensure even crisping on all sides. 6. Once finished, set the chickpeas aside to cool. 7. In the meantime, prepare the hummus dressing by whisking together hummus, tahini, lemon juice, salt, and olive oil in a small bowl. Adjust the seasoning to taste and set it aside. 8. Cut the romaine lettuce hearts in half or quarters, depending on their size, to create individual portions and place them on a large tray or individual plates. 9. Top each lettuce heart with equal amounts of cucumber, red onion, and roasted red peppers, and then add heaping spoonful of roasted chickpeas. 10. Finally, drizzle the hummus dressing over the top and sprinkle crumbled feta cheese as a garnish.

Per Serving: Calories 287; Fat 18.05g; Sodium 906mg; Carbs 25.49g; Fiber 6.7g; Sugar 7.62g; Protein 8.45g

Tomato Coconut Soup

Prep time: 15 minutes | Cook time: 30 minutes | Servings: 8

Ingredients:

4 tbsps. olive oil

1 tsp. salt plus more to taste

2 medium thinly sliced yellow onions

2 tsp. curry powder

1 tsp. ground coriander

1 tsp. red curry powder

5½ cups chicken broth

1 tsp. ground cumin

1 can diced tomatoes (15 ounces)

½ tsp. red pepper flakes

1 can diced tomatoes

1 can coconut milk (14 oz.)

Directions:

1. In a medium saucepan, heat the oil over medium heat. In a separate medium bowl, combine the salt and onions. 2. Cook the onions, stirring occasionally, for 10 to 12 minutes until fully softened and starting to brown. 3. Add the coriander, cumin, curry powder, and red pepper flakes, and stir continuously for 30 seconds. 4. Combine the tomatoes and their juices from the cans with five and a half cups of broth. Bring to a boil and cook for 15 minutes. 5. Use a hand blender to puree the mixture until smooth. If you do not have a hand blender, you can use a stand blender and puree the soup in three rounds. 6. Once the tomato soup is fully pureed, it can be served as is for a delicious, easy soup. 7. If desired, there are several options to customize the soup to your preferences. 8. For a creamier version, add some half and half and coconut milk. The soup pairs well with brown rice. 9. To add a bright flavor, serve the soup with lemon wedges.

Per Serving: Calories 381; Fat 21.55g; Sodium 1049mg; Carbs 7.15g; Fiber 1.6g; Sugar 4.48g; Protein 37.94g

Basil Beans and Carrot Soup

Prep time: 10 minutes | Cook time: 45 minutes | Servings: 5

Ingredients:

2 tbsp. olive oil

1 cup white onion (diced)

1½ tbsps. minced fresh garlic

2 tbsps. seasoning

1 large chopped carrot

1 diced celery stalk

1 medium chopped zucchini

1 can diced tomatoes (14 ounces)

1 can white beans (15 ounces)

3 tbsps. tomato paste

3 cups chopped spinach

6 cups vegetable broth (low sodium)

Sea salt

⅓ cup chopped fresh basil

pepper

Directions:

1. Preheat a saucepan over medium-high heat. When the oil is heated, add the onion and garlic and sauté until the onions become brownish and somewhat translucent, which usually takes about 3 minutes. 2. Next, add the celery and Land herb seasoning and cook for about a minute while checking to ensure that the herbs do not burn. Turn up the heat to high. 3. Combine the remaining ingredients in another medium-sized saucepan and bring them to a simmer. 4. Add a pinch of sea salt and freshly ground pepper, then reduce the heat to low, cover the pan, and let it cook for about half an hour. 5. Season with salt and ground pepper. Enjoy!

Per Serving: Calories 115; Fat 5.73g; Sodium 1918mg; Carbs 14.87g; Fiber 3.1g; Sugar 7.18g; Protein 2.26g

Sweet Potato and Blueberry Salad

Prep time: 20 minutes | Cook time: 20 minutes | Servings: 2

Ingredients:

For the sweet potatoes:

2 small sweet potato

1 tbsp. coconut oil

1 pinch salt and pepper

For the Dressing:

3 tbsps lemon juice

1 pinch pepper

1 pinch salt

1 tbsp. extra-virgin olive oil

For the Salad:

4 cups mixed greens

For Servings:

4 tbsps hummus

Fresh chopped parsley

1 cup raw blueberries

2 tbsps hemp seeds

1 medium ripe avocado

Directions:

1. Heat a large skillet over low heat. Season sweet potatoes with salt, pepper, and coconut oil, then add them to the skillet. 2. Cook the sweet potatoes until they are browned. 3. In a bowl, mix together lemon juice, salt, and pepper. Combine the mixed greens and sweet potatoes with the dressing. 4. Mix well, then serve.

Per Serving: Calories 458; Fat 29.3g; Sodium 662mg; Carbs 49g; Fiber 14g; Sugar 16g; Protein 8.6g

Chicken Pasta Soup

Prep time: 10 minutes | Cook time: 35 minutes | Servings: 8

Ingredients:

1 tbsp. Greek seasoning

1½ pounds chicken breasts (boneless and skinless)

1 tsp. pepper

4 thinly sliced green onions

1 tbsp. olive oil

1 minced garlic clove

¼ cup sun-dried tomatoes (chopped)

7 cups chicken broth (reduced-sodium)

¼ cup chicken broth

1½ tsps. minced fresh parsley

¼ cup sliced pitted Greek olives

½ tsp. dried basil

1 tbsp. drained capers

½ tsp. dried oregano

2 tbsp. lemon juice

1½ cups uncooked orzo pasta

Directions:

1. Coat the chicken with freshly ground black pepper and Greek seasoning. 2. Cook the chicken in oil in a Dutch oven until no longer pink; remove from heat and set aside. Cook garlic and green onions for 1 minute. 3. Add wine and scrape any browned bits from the bottom of the pan. 4. In a large mixing bowl, combine broth, onions, basil, olives, capers, oregano, and chicken. Increase heat to high and bring to a boil. 5. Reduce heat to low, cover, and simmer for 15 minutes. Bring back to a boil and add orzo. Cook for 8-10 minutes more or until the pasta is tender. 6. Add parsley and lemon juice at this stage.

Per Serving: Calories 547; Fat 26.35g; Sodium 1206mg; Carbs 10.61g; Fiber 2g; Sugar 1.38g; Protein 63.13g

Green Beans and Spinach Soup

Prep time: 5 minutes | Cook time: 25 minutes | Servings: 2

Ingredients:

3 tablespoons extra-virgin olive oil

1 large onion, diced

7 carrots, diced

¼ teaspoon ground turmeric

1 tablespoon coarse salt

10 cups water

8 oz. green beans, trimmed and cut into ½-inch pieces

3 packed cups baby spinach

3 tablespoons chopped fresh dill

3 lemons, halved

Directions:

1. Heat the olive oil in a large saucepan over medium heat. Add onions and cook, stirring occasionally, until they become soft, which should take about 6 minutes. 2. Next, add carrots, turmeric, and salt, and stir well. Add water to the pan and bring it to a boil. 3. Then, reduce heat and let it simmer for 30 minutes, or until the carrots become tender. Add beans and cook for an additional 2 minutes until they become tender. 4. To serve, place ⅓ of the spinach and dill in a bowl. 5. Ladle three cups of the hot soup over the greens, cover with a plate, let steep for 5 minutes. 6. Squeeze one lemon over the top and serve.

Per Serving: Calories 360; Fat 22.25g; Sodium 1702mg; Carbs 42.24g; Fiber 13.2g; Sugar 15.71g; Protein 6.65g

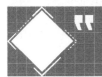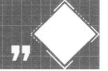

Beans and Grain Burgers

Prep time: 10 minutes | Cook time: 12 minutes | Servings: 2

Ingredients:

¼ cup bell peppers, finely diced

1 teaspoon oregano

1 teaspoon basil

Sea salt and cayenne pepper

¼ onion, diced

1½ cups garbanzo bean flour

1 teaspoon dill

1 tbsp. grapeseed oil

1½ cups cooked grains

Directions:

1. Heat the grapeseed oil in a pan and sauté the onion soft. 2. Transfer the onion to a bowl, add the remaining ingredients and toss well. 3. Form the mixture into patties and cook them in the pan for 4 minutes per side or until they are crispy.

Per Serving: Calories 833; Fat 19g; Sodium 49mg; Carbs 133g; Fiber 23g; Sugar 18g; Protein 38g

Salmon Watercress Pita Sandwich

Prep time: 10 minutes | Cook time: 0 minutes | Servings: 1

Ingredients:

2 tbsps. plain nonfat yogurt

2 tsps. lemon juice

2 tsps. fresh dill (chopped)

½ tsp. prepared horseradish

½ 6-inch whole-wheat pita bread

3 oz. flaked canned sockeye salmon (drained)

½ cup watercress

Directions:

1. Mix the yogurt, lemon juice, dill, and horseradish in a bowl; stir in salmon. 2. Put salad, salmon, and watercress in one side of the pita bread.

Per Serving: Calories 400; Fat 8.78g; Sodium 777mg; Carbs 55.11g; Fiber 6.9g; Sugar 4.3g; Protein 29.95g

Lemony Salmon with Fennel Seeds

Prep time: 8 minutes | Cook time: 10 minutes | Servings: 2

Ingredients:

2 medium salmon fillets, skinless and boneless	2 tbsp. olive oil
1 tbsp. fennel seeds	1 tbsp. lemon juice
	1 tbsp. water

Directions:

1. First, heat olive oil in a skillet, then add fennel seeds and toast them for a minute. 2. After that, add salmon fillets and lemon juice to the skillet, followed by water, and cook the fish over medium heat for 4 minutes on each side.

Per Serving: Calories 535; Fat 27.94g; Sodium 242mg; Carbs 2.04g; Fiber 1.2g; Sugar 0.19g; Protein 65.67g

Spicy Kale

Prep time: 5 minutes | Cook time: 15 minutes | Servings: 4

Ingredients:

¼ cup white onion, diced	¼ teaspoon sea salt
1 bunch of kale, fresh	1 teaspoon crushed red pepper
¼ cup red pepper, diced	2 tbsps grapeseed oil

Directions:

1. Start by washing the kale thoroughly and removing the stem, then cut the leaves into small pieces. Use a salad spinner to dry the kale leaves. 2. Heat a large skillet on high heat and add oil, onion, and red pepper. Cook for 3 minutes until the vegetables are starting to get soft. 3. Reduce the heat to low and add the kale leaves, toss to combine, and cover the skillet with a lid. Cook for 5 minutes. 4. Then, add the red pepper, toss to combine, cover the skillet again, and simmer for an additional 3 minutes until the vegetables are soft. 5. Serve immediately.

Per Serving: Calories 74; Fat 7g; Sodium 153mg; Carbs 2.7g; Fiber 0.9g; Sugar 1g; Protein 1g

Tasty Steak and Potatoes

Prep time: 15 minutes | Cook time: 45 minutes | Servings: 4

Ingredients:

4 potatoes, medium and thinly sliced

4 (4 oz.) cube steaks

1 large, thinly sliced onion

Salt and pepper according to taste

4 tsp margarine

Directions:

1. To prepare the meal, begin by preheating the oven to a temperature of 350°F. 2. Then, take four pieces of aluminum foil and lay them out. 3. Place a cube steak on each sheet of foil, and spread margarine over them before seasoning with pepper and salt. 4. Add sliced potatoes and onion rings over each steak and season again if desired. 5. Wrap the foil around the food and seal it tightly to create a packet. 6. Place the packets on a baking pan and bake in the preheated oven for 45 minutes or until the beef is fully cooked and the potatoes are soft. 7. Be careful when opening the packets as hot steam will be released.

Per Serving: Calories 649; Fat 11.63g; Sodium 564mg; Carbs 65.39g; Fiber 8.3g; Sugar 3.28g; Protein 68.38g

Zucchini Noodles with Avocado Sauce

Prep time: 10 minutes | Cook time: 5 minutes | Servings: 4

Ingredients:

4 large zucchinis, destemmed

4 avocados; pitted, peeled, sliced

4 cups basil leaves

48 cherry tomatoes, sliced

1½ teaspoon salt

1 cup walnuts, chopped

8 tbsps key lime juice

1 cup water

Directions:

1. To get zucchini noodles ready, remove the ends of each zucchini and use a spiralizer or vegetable peeler to make the noodles. 2. Keep them aside until needed. Then, blend avocado, basil, salt, and almonds in a blender with lime juice and water for 1-2 minutes until a thick sauce is formed. 3. Put the zucchini noodles in a large bowl, add the sauce along with tomatoes, and mix until the noodles are coated evenly. 4. Serve promptly.

Per Serving: Calories 500; Fat 43g; Sodium 889mg; Carbs 31g; Fiber 17.61g; Sugar 7.7g; Protein 9g

Garlicky Spinach, Tomatoes and White Beans

Prep time: 15 minutes | Cook time: 10 minutes | Servings: 2

Ingredients:

1 tablespoon olive oil	2 tablespoons water
4 small plum tomatoes, halved lengthwise	¼ teaspoon freshly ground black pepper
10 ounces frozen spinach, defrosted and squeezed of excess water	1 can white beans, drained
	Juice of 1 lemon
2 garlic cloves, thinly sliced	

Directions:

1. Heat oil in a large skillet over medium-high heat. Place the tomatoes with the cut side facing down and cook for 3 to 5 minutes. 2. Flip them and cook for an additional minute before transferring them to a plate. 3. Reduce the heat to medium and add spinach, garlic, water, and pepper to the skillet. Toss and cook for 2 to 3 minutes until the spinach is heated through. 4. Put the tomatoes back into the skillet, add white beans and lemon juice, and toss for 1 to 2 minutes until heated through.

Per Serving: Calories 497; Fat 4.52g; Sodium 172mg; Carbs 91.9g; Fiber 21.6g; Sugar 24g; Protein 29.91g

Tomato Basil Pasta

Prep time: 10 minutes | Cook time: 10 minutes | Servings: 6

Ingredients:

¾ teaspoon sea salt	1 oz. vegan pasta
½ cup extra-virgin olive oil	½ cup chopped fresh basil
1 small chopped cherry tomato basket	Salt & pepper as needed
2 finely chopped garlic cloves	

Directions:

1. Combine garlic, salt, and olive oil in a bowl, then add chopped cherry tomatoes and let the mixture rest for 30 minutes while stirring occasionally. 2. Cook the pasta as instructed, then drain it and save ½ cup of the pasta water. 3. Mix the pasta with the tomato mixture and add some pasta water as needed to adjust the consistency. 4. Serve with basil, salt, and pepper.

Per Serving: Calories 448; Fat g; Sodium 300mg; Carbs 58.1g; Fiber 3g; Sugar 3g; Protein 10g

Millet with Eggplant Chickpea Stew

Prep time: 10 minutes | Cook time: 35 minutes | Servings: 2

Ingredients:

1 cup millet

2 tbsps. ghee

Kosher salt

1 large Japanese eggplant

1 diced onion

Freshly ground black pepper

3 minced garlic cloves

1 (14-ounce) can tomatoes (puréed)

1 (14-ounce) can drained chickpeas

1 bunch cilantro

2 tbsps. harissa paste

Directions:

1. Combine millet, a pinch of salt, and 2 cups of water in a medium-sized saucepan. Simmer the mixture, cover it, and let it cook over low heat for 25 minutes. Once the millet is cooked, fluff it with a fork and let it cool. 2. While the millet is cooking, heat a shallow skillet over medium heat and melt 1 tablespoon of ghee or oil. Add eggplant, salt, and pepper and cook for about 10 minutes until the eggplant is golden brown and tender. 3. Add more ghee if required to prevent sticking. Place the cooked eggplant aside in a dish. 4. In the same skillet, add another tablespoon of ghee or oil and cook the onion until it becomes soft and golden brown (8-10 minutes). 5. Stir in garlic and cook for another 2 minutes. Add salt, pepper, tomatoes, chickpeas, and harissa, then lower the heat and add the eggplant. Let the mixture cook for 15 minutes. 6. Divide the cooked millet between two bowls and spoon the stew over it. Garnish with a few cilantro leaves and serve warm.

Per Serving: Calories 843; Fat 19.96g; Sodium 1277mg; Carbs 145.91g; Fiber 30.4g; Sugar 28.69g; Protein 27.71g

Cheese Prosciutto Corn Pizza

Prep time: 15 minutes | Cook time: 8 minutes | Servings: 4

Ingredients:

1-pound whole-wheat pizza dough

2 tbsps. olive oil (extra-virgin)

1 minced clove garlic

1 cup part-skim mozzarella cheese (shredded)

1 cup fresh corn kernels

1 oz. prosciutto (thinly sliced) torn into 1-inch pieces

1½ cups arugula

½ cup torn fresh basil

¼ tsp. ground pepper

Directions:

1. To prepare a grilled pizza, start by preheating the grill to medium-high. 2. Next, roll out the dough into an oval shape on a floured surface, and transfer it to a large baking sheet that has also been lightly floured. 3. In a small cup, mix together 1 tablespoon of oil and garlic. 4. Then, fire up the grill and place the dough on it along with the garlic oil, cheese, corn, and prosciutto. 5. Brush the grill rack with oil, and grill the dough for 1 to 2 minutes until it's puffed and lightly browned. 6. Flip the crust over and brush it with garlic oil. 7. Add the cheese, corn, and prosciutto on top, and grill for an additional 2 to 3 minutes until the cheese is melted and the bottom crust is lightly browned. 8. Once done, re-assemble the pizza and place it on the baking sheet. 9. Top with garlic, arugula, and pepper, and drizzle the remaining 1 tablespoon of oil over the top.

Per Serving: Calories 530; Fat 19.36g; Sodium 789mg; Carbs 70.2g; Fiber 3.3g; Sugar 1.7g; Protein 18.44g

Zucchini, Tofu and Green Beans

Prep time: 10 minutes | Cook time: 10 minutes | Servings: 4

Ingredients:

1-pound firm tofu	2 tbsps cold-pressed extra-virgin olive oil
3 medium-sized zucchinis	sea salt as needed
3 pieces tomatoes	pepper as needed
1-piece red bell pepper	½ tbsp. curry powder
1-piece green bell pepper	¼ tbsp. of ginger
½ pound green beans	fresh assorted selection of herbs
1 to 1½ cup fresh coconut milk	

Directions:

1. Slice the tofu and cut the zucchini, beans, tomatoes, and bell peppers into small pieces. 2. Heat some oil in a pan over medium heat, then cook the tofu for two to three minutes. 3. Next, stir-fry the zucchini, beans, and bell pepper for two to three minutes. 4. After adding the tomatoes, curry powder and coconut milk, let the dish cook for a little while. 5. Finally, season it with herbs, ginger, salt, and pepper and serve it with soba noodles or wild rice.

Per Serving: Calories 402; Fat 31g; Sodium 36mg; Carbs 17g; Fiber 6.71g; Sugar 6g; Protein 21.5g

Lemon-Garlic Artichokes

Prep time: 10 minutes | Cook time: 7 minutes | Servings: 2

Ingredients:

3 peeled and sliced garlic cloves	4 artichoke pieces
2 lemon pieces	1 tbsp. olive oil
1 tsp black pepper	1 tsp sea flavored vinegar

Directions:

1. Clean and soak the artichokes, then trim the stem to half an inch and remove the thorny tips and outer leaves. 2. Rub them with lemon and insert garlic slivers between the leaves. 3. Put the artichokes in a trivet basket in the Instant Pot and cook on high pressure for seven minutes. 4. Release the pressure naturally for 10 minutes, then transfer the artichokes to a cutting board to cool. Cut them in half lengthwise and remove the purple and white center. 5. Preheat the oven to 400°F and mix 1 and a half lemons with olive oil in a bowl, then pour over the artichoke halves and sprinkle with flavored vinegar and pepper. 6. Heat an iron skillet in the oven for 5 minutes, add a few teaspoons of oil, and place the marinated artichoke halves in the skillet. 7. Brush with the lemon and olive oil mixture and place quartered lemon slices between the halves. 8. Roast for 20-25 minutes until the artichokes are browned. 9. Serve and enjoy!

Per Serving: Calories 191; Fat 7.21g; Sodium 242mg; Carbs 29.56g; Fiber 14.2g; Sugar 2.75g; Protein 8.8g

Chickpea and Cilantro Tacos

Prep time: 20 minutes | Cook time: 20 minutes | Servings: 2

Ingredients:

1 tablespoon tamari	2 thinly sliced green onions
2 teaspoons garlic powder	½ sliced avocado
1½ cups drained & rinsed cooked chickpeas	1 tablespoon Sriracha hot sauce
½ teaspoon cumin	¼ shredded head cabbage
½ teaspoon onion powder	2 thinly sliced green onions
½ teaspoon paprika	Vegan sour cream
1 cup cilantro	Lime wedges

Directions:

1. To prepare the dish, in a small pan, combine chickpeas, onion powder, garlic, cumin, tamari, paprika, and hot sauce. 2. Heat the mixture over medium heat and remove from heat once it's cooked. 3. Warm the tortillas on the stove until slightly charred on the edges, and keep them warm in the pot. 4. Then, add the chickpea mixture, cabbage, cilantro, green onions, avocado, and vegan cream to each tortilla. 5. Finally, serve the dish warm with lime wedges.

Per Serving: Calories 362; Fat g; Sodium 1206mg; Carbs 52.61g; Fiber 14.51g; Sugar 0.8g; Protein 12g

Spiced Beef Burgers

Prep time: 10 minutes | Cook time: 12 minutes | Servings: 6

Ingredients:

1 medium-sized onion, chopped finely	½ teaspoon of ground cinnamon
4 teaspoons of minced fresh mint	½ teaspoon of salt
6 teaspoons of minced fresh parsley	A quarter teaspoon of ground nutmeg
1-2 garlic cloves chopped finely	1 pound of lean ground beef (90% lean)
3 quarter teaspoons of ground allspice	Lettuce leaves (optional)
3 quarter teaspoons of pepper	Tzaki sauce (optional)

Directions:

1. Combine the finely chopped onion, garlic, parsley, mint, pepper, salt, allspice, ground nutmeg, and ground beef in a mixing bowl, making sure to mix the spices thoroughly with the beef. 2. Shape the mixture into six oblong patties that are 4x2 inches in size. 3. Grill or broil the patties over medium heat, cooking each side for 4 to 6 minutes. 4. Use a thermometer to ensure that they are fully cooked, with a temperature of 160°F. 5. To serve, place the patties on lettuce leaves and serve with tzatziki sauce.

Per Serving: Calories 206; Fat 9.28g; Sodium 244mg; Carbs 9.19g; Fiber 1.2g; Sugar 5.29g; Protein 21g

Mushroom-Avocado Tacos

Prep time: 10 minutes | Cook time: 12 minutes | Servings: 4

Ingredients:

4 large Portobello mushrooms

2 medium red bell peppers, cored, sliced

4 medium green bell peppers, cored, sliced

2 medium white onions, peeled, sliced

⅔ teaspoon onion powder

⅔ teaspoon habanero seasoning

⅔ teaspoon cayenne pepper

1 key lime, juiced

2 tbsps grapeseed oil

2 medium avocados, peeled, pitted, sliced

8 tortillas, corn-free

Directions:

1. Prepare the mushrooms: Begin by cutting the mushrooms into pieces that are ⅓ inches in thickness after taking off the stems and gills. 2. Heat a large skillet on medium heat and add 1 tablespoon of oil. 3. Once heated, put in the onion and bell pepper and cook for about 2 minutes while stirring occasionally, or until the vegetables are tender-crisp. 4. Next, include the sliced mushrooms, add all the seasoning, mix everything together, and let it simmer for another 7 to 8 minutes until the vegetables are tender. 5. In the meantime, warm up the tortillas. 6. Assemble the tacos: Evenly distribute the cooked fajitas onto the center of each tortilla, add avocado on top, and sprinkle some lime juice. 7. Serve immediately.

Per Serving: Calories 375; Fat 23g; Sodium 70mg; Carbs 41g; Fiber 12g; Sugar 6.8g; Protein 7g

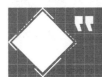

Avocado-Tuna Stuffed Cucumber Roll

Prep time: 8 minutes | Cook time: 0 minutes | Servings: 1

Ingredients:

¼ cucumber	2 tsp mustard in the yellow color (yellow or
1 can tuna	Dijon)
½ avocado	Salt and pepper (to taste)

Directions:

1. First, mix together tuna, avocado, and mustard in a bowl. Then, slice the cucumber into thin pieces that are one-fiftyth of an inch thick. 2. Before throwing away the cucumber slices, remove the seeds by either cutting them out with a knife or pushing them out with your fingers. 3. Next, stuff the cucumbers with the tuna mixture, making sure to fill the center completely. 4. Finally, add salt and pepper to taste and savor the dish!

Per Serving: Calories 334; Fat 17g; Sodium 700mg; Carbs 14.7g; Fiber 8g; Sugar 4.6g; Protein 35g

Lemony Pork Stew

Prep time: 15 minutes | Cook time: 50 minutes | Servings: 8

Ingredients:

2 lb. pork roast, sliced into cubes	2 teaspoons dried oregano
¼ cup chicken broth	2 teaspoons garlic powder
¼ cup lemon juice	

Directions:

1. Add the pork to the Instant Pot. Combine the remaining ingredients in a large bowl and pour the mixture over the pork. 2. Toss them to coat evenly and secure the pot. 3. Press the manual button and cook for 50 minutes at high pressure. Release the pressure naturally.

Per Serving: Calories 86; Fat 3.66g; Sodium 675mg; Carbs 2.21g; Fiber 0.3g; Sugar 1g; Protein 11.41g

White Fish and Potato Stew

Prep time: 10 minutes | Cook time: 22 minutes | Servings: 4

Ingredients:

2 tbsps. butter	1 tbsp. flour
1 chopped onion	1-pound boneless white fish
2 tbsps. olive oil (extra virgin)	Pepper to taste
1 round sliced carrot	½ tsp. smoked paprika
3 medium peeled and cut in bite sized	1-quart chicken broth
pieces potatoes	Salt to taste

Directions:

1. Heat the butter and olive oil in a skillet over medium heat, add the onions and carrots and cook for about 3 minutes until tender. 2. Then add flour and potatoes. Cook for an additional 1 minute. 3. Add the chicken broth and bring to a boil. Add the smoked paprika and fish. Cover the lid and cook over low heat, stirring frequently, cook for 15-20 minutes until potatoes are tender. 4. Flake the fish into tiny fragments and serve.

Per Serving: Calories 916; Fat 38g; Sodium 1826mg; Carbs 53g; Fiber 6.9g; Sugar 3.4g; Protein 86.99g

Pork with Tomatoes & Potatoes

Prep time: 15 minutes | Cook time: 22 minutes | Servings: 6

Ingredients:

1 lb. Lean pork, sliced into cubes	2 cups canned crushed tomatoes
1 onion, chopped	4 potatoes, cubed
2 carrots, sliced thinly	½ cup olive oil

Directions:

1. Turn the Instant Pot to sauté setting and add ½ cup of olive oil. Cook and stir the pork for 5 minutes. 2. Add the remaining and mix well. 3. Seal the pot and choose the manual setting. Cook for 17 minutes at high pressure. Release the pressure naturally.

Per Serving: Calories 386; Fat 22.38g; Sodium 878mg; Carbs 31.88g; Fiber 4.7g; Sugar 5.5g; Protein 16.68g

Spicy Flank Steak

Prep time: 15 minutes | Cook time: 16 minutes | Servings: 4

Ingredients:

2 green chili peppers

2 oz. beef flank steak

1 teaspoon salt

2 tablespoons olive oil

1 teaspoon apple cider vinegar

Directions:

1. Add olive oil to the skillet and place the flank steak in it. 2. Cook the steak for 3 minutes on each side, then season it with salt and apple cider vinegar. 3. Chop the chili peppers and add them to the skillet, and continue cooking the beef for another 10 minutes. 4. Remember to stir it occasionally.

Per Serving: Calories 41; Fat 3g; Sodium 603mg; Carbs 0.26g; Fiber 0.2g; Sugar 0.04g; Protein 3.11g

Tomato Farro Spaghetti

Prep time: 10 minutes | Cook time: 10 minutes | Servings: 4

Ingredients:

3 large tomatoes (about 2 pounds), cored and coarsely chopped

½ cup extra-virgin olive oil

2 garlic cloves, thinly sliced

½ teaspoon red-pepper flakes

½ cup fresh basil leaves, plus more for garnish

Coarse salt

10 oz. farro spaghetti

⅓ cup chopped Marcona almonds, for garnish

Directions:

1. Mix together tomatoes, oil, garlic, red pepper flakes, basil, and a small amount of salt in a bowl. 2. Leave the mixture at room temperature for 1 to 3 hours. Meanwhile, prepare spaghetti by cooking it in boiling salted water until it is cooked but still firm (al dente), as per package instructions. 3. Drain the spaghetti and put it back in the pot. 4. Combine the tomato sauce with the spaghetti and toss it together. When serving, decorate each dish with almonds and basil.

Per Serving: Calories 400; Fat 31.63g; Sodium 301mg; Carbs 26.45g; Fiber 5.9g; Sugar 4.56g; Protein 6.85g

Mustard Chicken Nuggets

Prep time: 8 minutes | Cook time: 20 minutes | Servings: 8

Ingredients:

1 cup all-purpose flour

4 tsp seasoned salt

1 teaspoon poultry seasoning

1 teaspoon ground mustard

1 teaspoon paprika

½ teaspoon pepper

2 pounds boneless and skinless chicken breasts

¼ cup canola oil

Directions:

1. In a wide and not so deep container, mix the initial six components. 2. Flatten the chicken to around ½ inch thickness and slice into pieces. 3. Take a few chicken pieces, cover them in the sauce, and place them on a serving platter. 4. Fry the chicken in canola oil in a frying pan over medium-high heat until it becomes crispy. 5. Serve and enjoy!

Per Serving: Calories 260; Fat 10g; Sodium 634mg; Carbs 13g; Fiber 1g; Sugar 0.3g; Protein 27g

Garlicky Balsamic Lamb Chops

Prep time: 10 minutes | Cook time: 20 minutes | Servings: 2

Ingredients:

Lamb chops, 8 ounces

2 tbsps Dijon mustard

2 tbsps Balsamic vinegar

1 tbsp. garlic, chopped

½ cup olive oil

1 tbsp. shredded fresh basil

Directions:

1. Place the lamb chops on a baking tray after drying them with a kitchen towel. 2. In a bowl, mix together Dijon mustard, balsamic vinegar, garlic, pepper, and basil. 3. Gradually whisk in the oil until the mixture is smooth. 4. Pour the marinade over the lamb chops and coat both sides. 5. Cover the chops and refrigerate for 1-4 hours. 6. Take the chops out of the refrigerator and let them sit for 30 minutes. 7. Preheat the grill to medium temperature and add oil to the grates. 8. Cook the lamb chops for 5-10 minutes on each side until both sides are browned. 9. The chops are cooked when the center registers 145°F. 10. Serve and enjoy!

Per Serving: Calories 678; Fat 62.37g; Sodium 267mg; Carbs 7.19g; Fiber 1.1g; Sugar 2.66g; Protein 24.16g

Buttermilk Chicken with Almonds and Yogurt Dressing

Prep time: 15 minutes | Cook time: 20 minutes | Servings: 6

Ingredients:

6 boneless, skinless chicken breasts (4 to 5 oz. each)	¼ cup finely chopped cornichons
1-quart buttermilk	2 teaspoons capers, rinsed and drained
4 sprigs sage	1 teaspoon finely grated lemon zest, plus 1 tablespoon fresh juice
4 garlic cloves, smashed	1 small head escarole, leaves torn
Coarse salt and freshly ground pepper	1 small head radicchio, leaves separated
1 cup plain Greek yogurt	4 radishes, thinly sliced
1 small shallot, minced	¼ cup sliced almonds, toasted

Directions:

1. The chicken should be left at room temperature for 30 minutes. 2. Reserve 3 tablespoons of buttermilk for the dressing and put the rest of the buttermilk, along with sage and garlic, in a Dutch oven or a large, heavy pot. 3. Season the chicken with salt and pepper and then submerge it in the buttermilk mixture in a single layer. 4. Heat the mixture over medium heat, stirring occasionally, until it starts to shimmer. Be careful not to let the buttermilk simmer, or it will curdle. 5. Poach the chicken, turning the pieces occasionally, until it is cooked through, which should take about 15 minutes. 6. Adjust the heat as needed to prevent the liquid from reaching a simmer. 7. Transfer the chicken to a dish and let it cool. Discard the poaching liquid. 8. In a separate bowl, mix together yogurt, shallot, cornichons, capers, lemon zest and juice, and the reserved buttermilk. Season the mixture with salt. 9. Arrange escarole and radicchio on a platter and then top them with chicken, radishes, and almonds. 10. Serve the dressing on the side.

Per Serving: Calories 267; Fat 9.98g; Sodium 959mg; Carbs 30.5g; Fiber 7.5g; Sugar 17g; Protein 16.2g

BBQ Shrimp with Kale and Cheese Couscous

Prep time: 15 minutes | Cook time: 30 minutes | Servings: 4

Ingredients:

1 cup chicken broth (low-sodium)

⅔ cup couscous (whole-wheat)

¼ tsp. poultry seasoning

⅓ cup Parmesan cheese (grated)

3 tbsp. olive oil (extra-virgin)

1 tbsp. butter

8 cups kale (chopped)

¼ cup barbecue sauce

1 large smashed clove garlic

¼ cup water

¼ tsp. salt

¼ tsp. red pepper (crushed)

1-pound raw shrimp (peeled and deveined)

Directions:

1. Combine poultry seasoning and broth in a medium-sized saucepan over medium-high heat. Once the mixture starts boiling, add couscous and remove the pan from heat. Cover it and let it sit for 5 minutes. 2. After that, use a fork to fluff the couscous and then mix in Parmesan cheese and butter by whisking with a fork. Keep the dish covered to maintain a warm temperature. 3. In the meantime, heat a tablespoon of oil in a big frying pan. Once the oil is hot, add the kale and cook for 1-2 minutes until it turns bright green, stirring occasionally. 4. Then add some water, cover the pan, and cook for around 3 minutes while stirring periodically until the kale becomes tender. 5. Lower the heat to medium-low. Create a well in the center of the kale and add garlic, a tablespoon of oil, and crushed red pepper. 6. Cook and stir occasionally for 15 seconds, then mix the garlic oil into the kale and sprinkle it with salt. 7. After that, transfer the kale to a large bowl and cover it to keep it warm. 8. Add one tablespoon of oil and the shrimp to the pan. Cook while stirring constantly for about 2 minutes, until the shrimp turns pink and curls. 9. Remove the pan from the heat and mix in the barbecue sauce. 10. Then, combine the shrimp, cabbage, and couscous together in a serving bowl.

Per Serving: Calories 435; Fat 21.46g; Sodium 1748mg; Carbs 18.13g; Fiber 1.7g; Sugar 6.72g; Protein 41g

Grilled Chicken with Cucumber-Radish Salad

Prep time: 10 minutes | Cook time: 30 minutes | Servings: 2

Ingredients:

¼ cup white-wine vinegar, plus more for drizzling (optional)

¼ cup water

1 teaspoon turbinado sugar

2 garlic cloves, smashed

1 small jalapeño chile, quartered (ribs and seeds removed for less heat, if desired)

Coarse salt and freshly ground pepper

1 cucumber, peeled and diced

5 radishes, very thinly sliced

8 oz. cherry tomatoes, halved

1 small red onion, finely diced

Canola or safflower oil, for grill

6 boneless, skinless chicken breast halves (4 to 5 oz. each)

1 cup fresh mint leaves, torn, plus whole leaves for garnish

Directions:

1. To make the vinegar mixture, combine vinegar, water, sugar, garlic, jalapeno, and salt in a small saucepan and bring it to a boil. 2. Remove it from the heat and let it stand for 15 minutes. 3. Then strain the mixture through a fine sieve and discard the solids. Allow it to cool completely. 4. Next, combine cucumber, radishes, tomatoes, and red onion in a bowl and pour in the vinegar mixture. Toss everything to coat. 5. Heat a grill (or grill pan) to medium-high and lightly oil the hot grates. Season the chicken with salt and pepper and grill it in batches until cooked through, around 6 to 7 minutes per side. 6. Transfer the chicken to a platter and let it stand for 10 minutes. Stir torn mint into the relish and season it with salt and pepper. 7. If desired, drizzle it with vinegar. Spoon the relish on top of the chicken and garnish it with mint leaves.

Per Serving: Calories 442; Fat 11.28g; Sodium 832mg; Carbs 67.15g; Fiber 18.5g; Sugar 44.58g; Protein 21.69g

Spinach, Tofu, and Brown Rice Bowl

Prep time: 10 minutes | Cook time: 75 minutes | Servings: 2

Ingredients:

6⅔ cups water

⅓ cup short-grain brown rice

Coarse salt and freshly ground pepper

½ package (14 oz.) firm tofu, drained, sliced into ¼-inch-thick pieces, and pressed

2 teaspoons tamari

1 tablespoon plus 1 teaspoon extra-virgin

olive oil, plus more for baking sheet

1 tablespoon plus 1 teaspoon grated peeled fresh ginger

2 garlic cloves, minced

1 cup packed baby spinach

2 scallions, trimmed and thinly sliced

2 tablespoons sesame seeds, toasted

Directions:

1. To cook the rice, combine ⅔ cup water, rice, and salt in a medium saucepan and bring to a boil. 2. Then reduce the heat, cover, and let it simmer for 40 to 50 minutes until the grains are tender and the water has been absorbed. 3. Remove from heat and let it stand for 10 minutes before fluffing it with a fork. 4. Preheat the oven to 350°F. Place tofu in a bowl and mix tamari and oil together. Season with salt and pepper, and drizzle the dressing over the tofu. Let it marinate for 20 minutes, tossing occasionally. 5. Arrange the tofu on an oiled baking sheet and bake for 10 minutes. Then flip the tofu and bake for an additional 30 minutes. 6. Meanwhile, fluff the rice again with a fork and add ginger, garlic, and the remaining 6 cups of water. 7. Bring to a boil and cook, stirring occasionally, until the broth has thickened, which takes about 25 minutes. Season with salt. 8. To serve, top the rice with tofu, spinach, scallions, and sesame seeds.

Per Serving: Calories 628; Fat 47.38g; Sodium 918mg; Carbs 25.87g; Fiber 9.5g; Sugar 6g; Protein 36.77g

Garlicky Pork Stew

Prep time: 10 minutes | Cook time: 10 hours | Servings: 4

Ingredients:

4 lb. pork shoulder (pork butt), skinless, boneless	1 onion , chopped
1 tsp salt	1 jalapeno , deseeded, chopped
1 tsp black pepper	4 cloves garlic, minced
Rub:	¾ cup juice from orange (2 oranges)
1 tbsp. dried oregano	1 tbsp. olive oil
2 tsp ground cumin	

Directions:

1. To prepare the pork, rinse and dry it, then season it with salt and pepper. 2. Next, make a rub by combining the specified ingredients and rub it all over the pork. 3. Place the seasoned pork in a slow cooker with the fat cap facing up, and add onions, jalapeños, minced garlic, and orange juice over the top. 4. Cook on low for 10 hours or on high for 7 hours until the pork is tender enough to shred. 5. After removing the pork from the slow cooker and letting it cool slightly, use two forks to shred it. 6. Optionally, skim off any excess fat from the remaining juices in the slow cooker and discard it. 7. If you have more than 2 cups of juice, reduce it down to about 2 cups. 8. Remember that the liquid will be salty and serves as seasoning for the pork, so do not strain out the soft onions, etc.

Per Serving: Calories 627; Fat 28.2g; Sodium 2626mg; Carbs 17.38g; Fiber 1.6g; Sugar 11.74g; Protein 78.6g

Lamb Chops with Mushrooms

Prep time: 10 minutes | Cook time: 35 minutes | Servings: 4

Ingredients:

8 lamb chops, about 2½ pounds

Salt, to taste

Freshly ground black pepper, to taste

1 tablespoon extra-virgin olive oil

¾ to 1 cup all-purpose flour

8 oz. mushrooms, sliced

6 green onions, sliced

4 cloves garlic, minced

1 tablespoon butter

1 cup beef broth

½ cup dry red wine

Directions:

1. Combine all the ingredients, then add salt and black pepper to the lamb chops. 2. Heat olive oil in a large skillet over medium-high heat. Lightly coat the lamb chops with flour and place them in the hot skillet, searing until well browned and turning them once. 3. Remove the lamb chops from the skillet and set them aside. Reduce the heat to medium, and then add mushrooms, green onions, garlic, and butter to the skillet. Stir the vegetables for 4 minutes. 4. Next, add beef broth and red wine to the skillet, simmer until the liquid has reduced by about one-third. 5. Finally, return the lamb chops to the skillet, cover it, and cook for about 15 to 20 minutes or until the lamb chops are cooked to your liking.

Per Serving: Calories 600; Fat 26.36g; Sodium 914mg; Carbs 27.48g; Fiber 1.8g; Sugar 1.93g; Protein 61.66g

Spicy White Fish and Tomato Soup

Prep time: 10 minutes | Cook time: 15 minutes | Servings: 4

Ingredients:

¼ cup water	⅓ cup sliced roasted red peppers
4 frozen white fish fillets, about 3-4 ounce each	2 tablespoons olive oil
	½ teaspoon salt
12 cherry tomatoes	A pinch of chili flakes
12-14 black olives	Garnish: chopped fresh parsley or basil
2 tablespoons marinated baby capers	(optional)

Directions:

1. Pour water into the Instant pot and then add the frozen fish fillets. Next, add the rest of the ingredients by spreading them around and on top of the fillets. 2. Sprinkle sea salt and chili flakes, followed by a drizzle of olive oil. 3. Close the lid and set the Instant Pot to "Manual" or "Pressure" Cook for four minutes under high pressure. After three beeps, the Instant Pot will start cooking. 4. Once the timer sounds, allow the pressure to release naturally for 7 to 8 minutes before doing a quick release to let the steam out. 5. Finally, open the lid, remove the cooked fish fillets carefully using a spatula, and place them on top of the soup. 6. Garnish with chopped parsley or basil, and serve.

Per Serving: Calories 1099; Fat 76g; Sodium 2922mg; Carbs 15g; Fiber 6g; Sugar 8.5g; Protein 87.5g

Lemony Mustard Pork

Prep time: 20 hours and 10 minutes | Cook time: 8 hours | Servings: 6

Ingredients:

5 pounds pork shoulder - boneless

¼ cup olive oil

2 tsps. oregano, dried

¼ cup lemon juice

2 tsps. mustard

2 tsps. mint, chopped

3 garlic cloves, minced

2 tsps. pesto sauce

Salt and black pepper to taste

Directions:

1. Mix together olive oil, lemon juice, oregano, mint, mustard, garlic, pecorino, salt, and pepper in a bowl using a whisk. 2. Use this mixture to marinate the pork for two hours, cover, and refrigerate for ten hours. 3. After that, flip the pork shoulder and leave it outside for ten more hours. 4. Then, transfer the marinated pork and the prepared juices to a slow cooker and cook it covered on low for eight hours. 5. Finally, slice the pork, divide it between plates, and serve.

Per Serving: Calories 1104; Fat 76g; Sodium 639mg; Carbs 3.15g; Fiber 0.5g; Sugar 1.49g; Protein 95g

Chicken Mushroom Meatloaf

Prep time: 15 minutes | Cook time: 45 minutes | Servings: 8

Ingredients:

5½ pounds lean ground chicken	1 teaspoon thyme
1 medium onion	¼ cup fresh basil
1 green pepper	¼ cup fresh parsley
½ cups zucchini	Salt and pepper, to taste
½ cups broccoli	4 egg whites.
2 stalks celery	2 cups rolled organic oats in the organic form
1 ounce chopped mushrooms	1 bulb garlic, minced

Directions:

1. To prepare the vegetables, spray a skillet with cooking spray and add onions, peppers, zucchini, broccoli, celery, and mushrooms. 2. Cook them over medium heat for a few minutes, then add garlic. 3. Once the vegetables are almost done, turn off the heat and let them cool for about 5 minutes. 4. Combine the cooked vegetables with other ingredients in a big bowl and stir. 5. Grease a baking dish before pouring the batter in and baking it for 40 minutes at 425°F. 6. After taking it out of the oven, let it cool for 45 minutes before serving. 7. Cut the chicken into 8 pieces before eating.

Per Serving: Calories 600; Fat 27.8g; Sodium 395mg; Carbs 26g; Fiber 6g; Sugar 8g; Protein 64g

Cheese Spinach Stuffed Chicken Breasts

Prep time: 15 minutes | Cook time: 30 minutes | Servings: 8

Ingredients:

½ cup feta cheese (crumbled)	2 minced cloves garlic
½ cup fresh spinach (chopped)	¼ tsp. salt
½ cup roasted red bell peppers (chopped)	4 chicken breasts (boneless, skinless)
¼ cup Kalamata olives, pitted and quartered	½ tsp. pepper (ground)
1 tbsp. fresh flat-leaf parsley (chopped)	1 tbsp. lemon juice
1 tbsp. fresh basil (chopped)	1 tbsp. olive oil (extra-virgin)

Directions:

1. To begin, preheat the oven to 400°F. 2. Next, combine parsley, roasted red peppers, feta, spinach, basil, olives, and garlic in a medium bowl. 3. Use a small knife to make a horizontal cut through the thickest part of each chicken breast to create a pocket, and then stuff each pocket with about ⅓ cup of the feta mixture. 4. Secure the pockets with wooden picks and season the chicken with salt and pepper. 5. Heat oil in an oven-safe skillet over medium-high heat and place the stuffed chicken breasts in the pan with the top side down. 6. Cook for approximately 2 minutes or until golden, then carefully flip the chicken and place the skillet in the oven. 7. Bake for 20-25 minutes and drizzle lemon juice evenly over the chicken before serving.

Per Serving: Calories 298; Fat 17.58g; Sodium 283mg; Carbs 1.67g; Fiber 0.3g; Sugar 0.74g; Protein 31.85g

Simple Boiled Unshelled Peanuts

Prep time: 5 minutes | Cook time: 7-10 hours | Servings: 32

Ingredients:

2 pounds raw peanuts in the shell

7 tbsps salt

Water, to cover peanuts

Directions:

1. Thoroughly wash unshelled peanuts with cold water. 2. Then, soak them overnight in water with 7 tablespoons of salt in your slow cooker. 3. The next day, cook the peanuts on low heat for 7 to 10 hours until they are soft. 4. The boiled peanuts should have soft and pliable shells, not crispy and rigid. 5. Once drained, allow the peanuts to cool for ten minutes before serving. 6. Remove their shells before eating and store any leftovers in the refrigerator or freezer. 7. Reheat before serving again.

Per Serving: Calories 160; Fat 13.8g; Sodium 3mg; Carbs 4.7g; Fiber 2.4g; Sugar 1g; Protein 7g

Minty Tomato and Avocado Rolls

Prep time: 10 minutes | Cook time: 15 minutes | Servings: 4

Ingredients:

1 cup chopped trimmed watercress

½ mashed ripe avocado

1 carrot

10 fresh mint leaves

Cabbage leaves

Directions:

1. Combine 1 cup of trimmed and chopped watercress with half of a mashed ripe avocado, one peeled carrot julienned, and ten fresh mint leaves. 2. Add coarse salt to taste. 3. Divide the mixture evenly between halves of a cabbage leaf, top with another julienned carrot and ten fresh mint leaves, then roll up to enclose. 4. Serve immediately.

Per Serving: Calories 100; Fat 5g; Sodium 22mg; Carbs 13.76g; Fiber 2.9g; Sugar 8.78g; Protein 1.34g

Spiced Nuts Mix

Prep time: 15 minutes | Cook time: 2 hours | Servings: 22

Ingredients:

1 cup unsalted cashews

1 cup unsalted almonds

1 cup unsalted pecans

1 cup unsalted, shelled pistachios

½ cup maple syrup

⅓ cup melted coconut oil

1 teaspoon ground ginger

½ teaspoon sea salt

½ teaspoon cinnamon

¼ teaspoon ground cloves

¼ teaspoon cayenne pepper

Directions:

1. To cook the nuts, first spray the crock with nonstick cooking spray. 2. Then, mix in the other ingredients with the nuts and ensure they are evenly distributed. 3. Place a piece of paper towel or a thin dishtowel beneath the lid before covering the crock. 4. Cook on low heat for one hour, stirring the nuts afterwards. 5. Repeat stirring after two hours and then spread the nuts out on a parchment paper-covered cookie sheet. 6. Let them cool for an hour before serving or storing leftovers in an airtight jar for up to three weeks.

Per Serving: Calories 194; Fat 16.4g; Sodium 55mg; Carbs 10.4g; Fiber 2g; Sugar 5.6g; Protein 4g

Coconut and Nuts Trail Mix

Prep time: 5 minutes | Cook time: 0 minutes | Servings: 2

Ingredients:

½ cup pistachios

½ cup dried apricots

½ cup toasted unsweetened coconut flakes

½ cup chopped almonds

Directions:

1. Mix ½ cup each of shelled unsalted pistachios, chopped unsweetened dried apricots, toasted unsweetened coconut flakes, and chopped toasted almonds in a bowl. 2. The trail mix can be stored in an airtight container at room temperature for up to 2 weeks. 3. This recipe yields 2 cups of trail mix.

Per Serving: Calories 481; Fat 31.55g; Sodium 64mg; Carbs 44.79g; Fiber 10.5g; Sugar 28.53g; Protein 12.86g

Crispy Flaxseed Crackers

Prep time: 5 minutes | Cook time: 30 minutes | Servings: 1

Ingredients:

1 cup ground flaxseed	1 teaspoon cayenne pepper
1 teaspoon powdered garlic	½ cup water
1 teaspoon powdered onion	

Directions:

1. Mix all the ingredients in a suitable bowl and add water to form a dough. Let it rest for 10 minutes. 2. Spread the dough on a baking sheet covered with parchment paper, and use another parchment paper to roll it into a thin rectangle. 3. Cut the dough into squares using a sharp knife and place them on a baking sheet lined with parchment paper. 4. Bake at 400°F for 30 minutes, rotating halfway through to make sure both sides are crispy.

Per Serving: Calories 921; Fat 71g; Sodium 57mg; Carbs 53.7g; Fiber 47g; Sugar 3g; Protein 31.7g

Crispy Beet Chips

Prep time: 10 minutes | Cook time: 15 minutes | Servings: 4

Ingredients:

8 medium to large beets	1 tbsp. flaked sea salt
Olive oil	1 tbsp. dried chives

Directions:

1. First, prepare the beets by removing the greens and roots, then washing them thoroughly and slicing them very thinly using a mandoline or a sharp knife. 2. Preheat the oven to 400°F and lightly coat a baking sheet with a small amount of olive oil. 3. Arrange the sliced beets on the sheet in a single layer, making sure they don't overlap, and bake them on the bottom rack of the oven for 10-15 minutes until they are crispy. 4. While the beets are baking, mix salt and dried chives in a small cup. 5. Sprinkle the chive salt on the chips when they come out of the oven, and let them cool and crisp up on the pan before transferring them to a cooling rack. 6. Repeat the process with the remaining beet slices.

Per Serving: Calories 101; Fat 3.66g; Sodium 1872mg; Carbs 15.71g; Fiber 4.6g; Sugar 11g; Protein 2.66g

Beet-White Bean Hummus

Prep time: 10 minutes | Cook time: 10 minutes | Servings: 2

Ingredients:

1 small beet

1 cup white beans

2 tablespoons lemon juice

1 chopped garlic clove

1 tablespoon olive oil

Salt

Pepper

Directions:

1. Before cooking, heat the oven to 425°F. Cook one small beet by roasting it and remove the skin by rubbing it off. 2. After chopping the beet, blend it together with 1 cup of cooked white beans (which have been drained and rinsed), 2 tablespoons of fresh lemon juice, 1 chopped garlic clove, and 1 tablespoon of extra-virgin olive oil until well combined. Add coarse salt and freshly ground pepper to taste. 3. The hummus can be kept in an airtight container in the refrigerator for up to three days. 4. Before serving, add more pepper and enjoy with crudités.

Per Serving: Calories 442; Fat 3.25g; Sodium 511mg; Carbs 82g; Fiber 18.5g; Sugar 19.28g; Protein 24.68g

Peanut Butter Banana Yogurt Bowls

Prep time: 5 minutes | Cook time: 30 seconds | Servings: 4

Ingredients:

4 cups vanilla Greek yogurt

2 medium sliced bananas

¼ cup creamy natural peanut butter

¼ cup flax seed meal

1 teaspoon nutmeg

Directions:

1. Divide the yogurt into four equal portions and place them in separate bowls. Then, add banana slices to each bowl. 2. Take a cup that is safe to use in the microwave, put peanut butter in it, and heat it in the microwave for thirty seconds. 3. After that, pour one tablespoon of the melted peanut butter over the bananas in each bowl. 4. When you're ready to serve, sprinkle some ground nutmeg and flax seed meal on top of the bowls.

Per Serving: Calories 171; Fat 9.16g; Sodium 75mg; Carbs 19.49g; Fiber 2.3g; Sugar 9.9g; Protein 6.33g

Cheese Pasta with Crab Rangoon Dip

Prep time: 10 minutes | Cook time: 25 minutes | Servings: 2

Ingredients:

For the Pasta Chips:

8 oz. dried farfalle pasta

1 ounce finely grated Parmesan cheese (about ½ cup)

3 tablespoons neutral oil, such as canola or

grapeseed

1 teaspoon garlic powder

1 teaspoon red pepper flakes

Cooking spray

For the Crab Rangoon Dip (Optional):

1 small scallion

4 oz. whipped cream cheese

4 oz. lump crab meat, drained

⅛ teaspoon kosher salt

⅛ teaspoon freshly ground black pepper

¼ cup Thai sweet chili sauce (optional)

Directions:

1. To begin, boil a large pot of salted water and cook 8 oz. of farfalle pasta according to the instructions until tender. 2. Meanwhile, preheat the oven to 400°F (or an air fryer to 350°F) and grate 1 ounce of Parmesan cheese. 3. Once the pasta is ready, drain it and transfer it to a large bowl, then add 3 tablespoons of neutral oil and toss to coat. 4. Add the grated cheese, 1 teaspoon of garlic powder, and 1 teaspoon of red pepper flakes, and toss again to coat. 5. If using the oven, coat a rimmed baking sheet with cooking spray and arrange the pasta in a single layer, making sure the noodles aren't touching. 6. If using the air fryer, coat the basket with cooking spray and add the pasta in a single layer, working in batches if necessary. 7. Bake for 18 to 25 minutes or air fry for 10 to 12 minutes, until the pasta is crispy and golden. Let it cool to room temperature. 8. To make the crab Rangoon dip, mince 1 small scallion and place it in a medium bowl. Add 4 oz. of whipped cream cheese, 4 oz. of drained lump crab meat, ⅛ teaspoon of kosher salt, and ⅛ teaspoon of black pepper, and stir until combined. 9. Serve the pasta chips with the crab Rangoon dip and ¼ cup of Thai sweet chili sauce on the side, if desired.

Per Serving: Calories 724; Fat 38g; Sodium 460mg; Carbs 69g; Fiber 17.1g; Sugar 2.77g; Protein 32.81g

Herbed Potato Chips

Prep time: 10 minutes | Cook time: 20 minutes | Servings: 2

Ingredients:

¼ cup olive oil

2 cloves garlic, thinly sliced

2 sprigs fresh thyme, bruised

2 sprigs fresh oregano, bruised

1 medium russet potato

1 small, sweet potato

¼ teaspoon coarse sea salt or table salt

Directions:

1. Heat oil, garlic, thyme, and oregano in a small saucepan over medium-low heat for 15 minutes. 2. If the garlic starts to bubble, reduce the heat to low. Remove from heat and let stand at room temperature until cool. 3. Remove the garlic and herb sprigs from the oil, and set aside 2 tablespoons of the oil. 4. Preheat the oven to 425°F and line two large baking sheets with parchment paper. Brush the paper with some of the herb-infused oil. 5. Scrub the potatoes and slice them using a mandoline to ⅛ inch thickness. 6. Arrange the russet potato slices in a single layer on one of the prepared baking sheets and arrange the sweet potato slices in a single layer on the other prepared sheet. 7. Brush the tops of the potato slices with the remaining herb-infused oil. Bake the potato slices on a baking sheet one sheet at a time for 24 to 26 minutes, or until they turn golden brown. 8. Flip the slices over halfway through baking. Check the potatoes frequently during the last 2 to 3 minutes of baking as they may brown at different rates. 9. Once a slice has browned nicely, transfer it onto a clean piece of parchment paper and lightly sprinkle it with salt. 10. Serve immediately.

Per Serving: Calories 390; Fat 27.24g; Sodium 333mg; Carbs 34.93g; Fiber 4.4g; Sugar 3.47g; Protein 3.76g

Almonds and Cheese Stuffed Figs

Prep time: 15 minutes | Cook time: 3 minutes | Servings: 12

Ingredients:

4 oz. herbed goat cheese	2 tsp balsamic vinegar
12 fresh figs, halved	1 tbsp. honey
24 almonds	

Directions:

1. Before starting, preheat the oven to high broil heat. 2. Then, take the fig halves and place them on a baking sheet, with the cut side facing up. 3. Next, add half a teaspoon of goat cheese on each half, followed by gently pressing one almond on top of each fig and pushing the cheese into the fig. 4. Broil the figs in the preheated oven for two to three minutes until the cheese becomes soft and the almonds turn a deep brown color. 5. Once done, remove them from the oven and let them cool for five minutes. 6. Afterward, transfer the figs onto a serving platter and drizzle them with balsamic vinegar and honey. 7. Before serving, make sure to heat the dish.

Per Serving: Calories 100; Fat 5.57g; Sodium 49mg; Carbs 9.22g; Fiber 1.4g; Sugar 7g; Protein 4.41g

Lemony Roasted Chickpeas

Prep time: 5 minutes | Cook time: 30 minutes | Servings: 2

Ingredients:

2 cans chickpeas (15 ounces)

2 teaspoons red wine vinegar

2 tablespoons olive oil (extra virgin)

½ teaspoon black pepper (cracked)

2 teaspoons fresh lemon juice

1 teaspoon dried oregano

1 teaspoon kosher salt

½ teaspoon garlic powder

Directions:

1. First, preheat your oven to 425°F and line a baking sheet with parchment paper. 2. After draining, cleaning, and drying the chickpeas, place them in a single layer on the baking sheet. 3. Roast them for 10 minutes, then turn them over with a spatula to make sure they cook evenly and roast for another 10 minutes. 4. In a large mixing bowl, mix the remaining ingredients together, then carefully toss the hot chickpeas in the mixture until they are fully coated. 5. Place the coated chickpeas back on the baking sheet and roast for another 10 minutes, checking regularly to make sure they don't overcook and burn. 6. Finally, allow the chickpeas to cool completely before serving.

Per Serving: Calories 479; Fat 20.57g; Sodium 1787mg; Carbs 58.77g; Fiber 16.7g; Sugar 10.32g; Protein 18.11g

Almond-Walnuts Crackers

Prep time: 15 minutes | Cook time: 15 minutes | Servings: 5

Ingredients:

2 tbsp. finely chopped walnuts	1 ½ tsp flaxseed meal
1 ½ tsp olive oil	2 tbsp. water
1 cup of almond flour	½ tsp salt

Directions:

1. To start, preheat your oven to 350°F and line a baking sheet with parchment paper. 2. In a mixing bowl, combine the walnuts, almond flour (or almond meal and pumpkin seed meal), salt, and flaxseed meal. 3. Mix in the olive oil and water until the dough becomes sticky and holds together. 4. Next, place the dough on the prepared baking sheet and cover with a second sheet of parchment paper. 5. Use a rolling pin to stretch the dough into a 1/16-inch wide rectangle. 6. Remove the top parchment paper and cut the dough into 1-inch squares using a pizza cutter. 7. Hold the dough together while cutting it into squares. 8. Bake in the preheated oven for 15 minutes until the outer edges are browned. 9. Let the crackers cool on the baking sheet before breaking them into squares.

Per Serving: Calories 32; Fat 3.16g; Sodium 233mg; Carbs 0.55g; Fiber 0.4g; Sugar 0g; Protein 0.93g

Delicious Hoisin Button Mushrooms

Prep time: 10 minutes | Cook time: 5-6 hours | Servings: 10

Ingredients:

24 ounces whole button mushrooms, trimmed

1 small sweet onion, halved, sliced

¼ cup water

3 cloves garlic, minced

2 tbsps gluten-free soy sauce or Bragg's

liquid aminos

1 tbsp. smooth natural peanut butter

1 teaspoon rice wine vinegar

1 teaspoon sesame oil

¼ teaspoon crushed red pepper

Directions:

1. To cook the dish, first, apply nonstick cooking spray on the crock. Then, put mushrooms and onions into the crock. 2. In a big mixing bowl, mix water, garlic, rice wine vinegar, soy sauce, peanut butter, sesame oil, and crushed red pepper together, and pour this mixture over the mushrooms and onions. 3. It is essential to pour the mixture over the vegetables. Cover and cook the dish on low heat for 5 to 6 hours. 4. Once the cooking is done, gently fold the mushrooms into the sauce before removing them with a slotted spoon for serving. 5. Serve the mushrooms on toothpicks and, if desired, add green onion and sesame seeds as a garnish.

Per Serving: Calories 228; Fat 1.8g; Sodium 124mg; Carbs 54.9g; Fiber 8.3g; Sugar 3.4g; Protein 7.6g

Nutty Cranberry Oats

Prep time: 10 minutes | Cook time: 2-3 hours | Servings: 12

Ingredients:

5 cups gluten-free Cheerios	¼ cup melted coconut oil
3 cups gluten-free Honey Nut Cheerios	¼ cup honey
1 cup gluten-free oats	½ teaspoon cinnamon
1 cup dried cranberries	½ teaspoon salt
2 cups unsweetened shredded coconut	1 teaspoon coconut oil
2 cups raw almonds, chopped	1 teaspoon vanilla extract

Directions:

1. Apply cooking spray to the slow cooker and add Cheerios, Honey Nut Cheerios, gluten-free oats, cranberries, coconut, and almonds evenly throughout. In a mixing bowl, mix coconut oil, honey, cinnamon, salt, and vanilla. 2. Use a rubber spatula to gently toss the cereal in the slow cooker after adding the mixture to ensure it is evenly coated. 3. Cover the slow cooker with a lid and cook on low heat setting for 2-3 hours, stirring the mixture every 45 minutes to prevent burning. 4. After cooking, let the mixture cool on a baking sheet lined with parchment paper for an hour before serving or storing in an airtight container at room temperature for up to 3 weeks.

Per Serving: Calories 252; Fat 10g; Sodium 230mg; Carbs 42.5g; Fiber 3.5g; Sugar 16g; Protein 3.7g

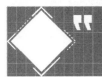

Chapter 7 Dessert Recipes

Nutty Protein Truffles

Prep time: 10 minutes | Cook time: 0 minutes | Servings: 20

Ingredients:

½ cup honey peanut butter, roasted

½ cup ricotta cheese, whole-milk

⅓ cup dry roasted peanut, chopped

2 tbsp. peanut butter-flavored syrup, sugar-free

2 scoops of vanilla protein powder

1 tsp vanilla extract

1 pinch of salt

2 pockets of stevia-erythritol sweetener

Directions:

1. Mix together ricotta cheese, vanilla extract, and maple syrup in a bowl, using a hand mixer to blend them well. 2. Then, add sweetener, salt, and protein powder and continue to mix until the mixture becomes smooth. 3. Shape the mixture into small balls of one-inch size and coat them with peanut butter. 4. Finally, refrigerate the balls until you're ready to serve.

Per Serving: Calories 91; Fat 7.32g; Sodium 511mg; Carbs 4g; Fiber 0.1g; Sugar 2.87g; Protein 2.7g

Simple Whipped Cream

Prep time: 10 minutes | Cook time: 10 minutes | Servings: 1

Ingredients:

1 cup of Aquafaba

¼ cup of Agave Syrup

Directions:

1. Mix maple syrup and quafa in a bowl and use a hand mixer for 10-15 minutes or a stand mixer for 5-10 minutes at high speed. 2. Once mixed, you can enjoy your own whipped cream as a snack!

Per Serving: Calories 112; Fat 5.12g; Sodium 125mg; Carbs 15.8g; Fiber 0.7g; Sugar 9g; Protein 0.73g

Strawberry-Applesauce Ice Cream

Prep time: 10 minutes | Cook time: 0 minutes | Servings: 4

Ingredients:

3 cups of homemade applesauce	3 tbsp. agave nectar
1 cup strawberries, frozen	2 tbsp. homemade hemp sea moss milk
¼ cup sea moss gel	½ small squeezed key lime

Directions:

1. Put all the ingredients in a blender and blend until the mixture becomes thick and smooth. Adjust the taste to your liking. 2. Pour the mixture into a glass container and even it out. 3. You can either serve it immediately while it's soft, or freeze it for 2-4 hours, covered, to make it more solid. 4. Before serving, let it thaw for 2 to 5 minutes. You can store the ice cream in the freezer for up to two weeks. Bon appétit!

Per Serving: Calories 104; Fat 0.57g; Sodium 13mg; Carbs 26.46g; Fiber 3.5g; Sugar 19.73g; Protein 0.99g

Yogurt Pumpkin Parfait with Nuts

Prep time: 30 minutes | Cook time: 0 minutes | Servings: 6

Ingredients:

1 can pumpkin puree (15 ounces)	2 tablespoons molasses
3-4 tbsp. mascarpone cheese	2 teaspoons ground cinnamon
1 and a quarter cup Greek yogurt (low-fat)	Chocolate chips
1 tsp. vanilla extract	Pinch of nutmeg
2½ tablespoons brown sugar	Walnuts or hazelnuts (chopped)

Directions:

1. Mix together yogurt, pumpkin puree, and other ingredients except for nuts and chocolate chips in a large mixing bowl until smooth. 2. Adjust the flavor to your preference and mix again. Divide the mixture into small goblets or mason jars and refrigerate for at least 30 minutes or overnight. 3. To serve, add molasses, chocolate chips, and chopped nuts on top of each serving. 4. Enjoy your delicious creation!

Per Serving: Calories 124; Fat 3.77g; Sodium 178mg; Carbs 19g; Fiber 1.1g; Sugar 15g; Protein 4.65g

Coconut Mint Mousse

Prep time: 10 minutes | Cook time: 0 minutes | Servings: 4

Ingredients:

1½ cups raw coconut meat, chopped	12 drops liquid stevia
1 tablespoon fresh mint leaves	¼ cup almond butter
1 tablespoon chia seeds	1 teaspoon organic vanilla extract
1¼ cups unsweetened almond milk	3 tablespoons fresh raspberries

Directions:

1. Put all the ingredients except for the raspberries in a blender and blend until the mixture becomes creamy and smooth. 2. Afterwards, pour the mixture into serving bowls and chill them in the refrigerator before serving. 3. Finally, add raspberries on top of the chilled mixture for decoration and serve.

Per Serving: Calories 281; Fat 21.07g; Sodium 96mg; Carbs 22.23g; Fiber 6.3g; Sugar 13.35g; Protein 5.5g

Grilled Peaches with Yogurt Honey Dressing

Prep time: 10 minutes | Cook time: 10 minutes | Servings: 4

Ingredients:

4 peaches (ripe)	1 cup Greek yogurt
6 tbsps. honey	1 tsp. cinnamon

Directions:

1. Cut peaches in half and place them with the cut side facing down on the grill. Grill them for about 4 to 5 minutes on each side or until they become soft. 2. As you grill, mix yogurt and four teaspoons of honey in a bowl. 3. After grilling, take the peaches off the grill and put a tablespoon of the yogurt mixture on each peach half. 4. Finally, add a drizzle of honey and sprinkle some cinnamon on top. 5. Repeat the process for the remaining peach slices. 6. Serve and enjoy!

Per Serving: Calories 193; Fat 2.37g; Sodium 30mg; Carbs 43.64g; Fiber 2.7g; Sugar 41.32g; Protein 3.61g

Classic Banana-Almond Cake

Prep time: 15 minutes | Cook time: 45 minutes | Servings: 8

Ingredients:

4 ripe bananas in chunks	1 tsp cinnamon
3 tbsp. honey or maple syrup	1 tsp baking powder
1 tsp pure vanilla extract	1 pinch of salt
½ cup almond milk	⅓ cup of almonds finely chopped
¾ cup of self-rising flour	Almond slices for decoration

Directions:

1. To start, heat the oven to 400°F. Grease a cake mold and keep it aside. 2. Take a bowl, add bananas and mash them with a fork. Add honey, vanilla, and almond to it and mix them well. 3. In a separate bowl, mix flour, cinnamon, baking powder, salt, and broken almonds with a spoon. 4. Combine the flour mixture with the banana mixture and stir until everything is well combined. 5. Transfer the mixture to the greased cake mold and sprinkle with sliced almonds. Bake for 40-45 minutes or until the toothpick inserted comes out clean. 6. Once done, take it out of the oven and let the cake cool down completely. 7. Cut the cake into slices and store them in an airtight container or tin foil in the refrigerator for up to a week.

Per Serving: Calories 139; Fat 3.33g; Sodium 240mg; Carbs 26.72g; Fiber 1.8g; Sugar 11.8g; Protein 1.83g

Prosciutto Wrapped Plums

Prep time: 5 minutes | Cook time: 0 minutes | Servings: 8

Ingredients:

2 ounces prosciutto, cut into 16 pieces	A pinch of red pepper flakes, crushed
1 tbsp. chives, chopped	3 Plums, quartered

Directions:

1. To present the dish, take a quarter of a plum and wrap it with a slice of prosciutto. 2. Then, put it on a plate and sprinkle some chive and red pepper flakes over it.

Per Serving: Calories 34; Fat 1.31g; Sodium 66mg; Carbs 4.76g; Fiber 0.4g; Sugar 3.88g; Protein 1.39g

Chocolate Banana Smoothie Bowls

Prep time: 10 minutes | Cook time: 0 minutes | Servings: 4

Ingredients:

4 large frozen bananas, peeled and sliced

2 cups unsweetened soy milk

⅓ cup cacao powder

2 scoops of vegan unsweetened protein powder

Directions:

1. Place all the ingredients into a high-speed blender and blend until the mixture becomes creamy. 2. Then, pour the mixture into three serving bowls and add your preferred topping. 3. Serve right away.

Per Serving: Calories 298; Fat 6.62g; Sodium 220mg; Carbs 47.53g; Fiber 7.2g; Sugar 27.92g; Protein 19.11g

Blueberry and Dates Chia Pudding

Prep time: 20 minutes | Cook time: 0 minutes | Servings: 3

Ingredients:

⅔ cup unsweetened almond milk

2 cups frozen blueberries

½ of frozen banana, peeled and sliced

5 large soft dates, pitted and chopped

½ cup chia seeds

Directions:

1. Combine all ingredients, except for chia seeds, in a food processor and blend until the mixture becomes smooth. 2. Then, move the mixture to a bowl, add chia seeds, and mix well. 3. Refrigerate the mixture for half an hour, stirring it every 5 minutes.

Per Serving: Calories 153; Fat 2.88g; Sodium 40mg; Carbs 32.94g; Fiber 6.1g; Sugar 23.32g; Protein 2.05g

Strawberry Chocolate Tofu Mousse

Prep time: 2 hours | Cook time: 0 minutes | Servings: 6

Ingredients:

1-pound firm tofu, drained	10-15 drops liquid stevia
¼ cup unsweetened almond milk	1 tablespoon organic vanilla extract
2 tablespoons cacao powder	¼ cup fresh strawberries

Directions:

1. Put all the ingredients, except the strawberries, into a blender and blend them until you get a smooth and creamy mixture. 2. Then, pour the mixture into bowls and refrigerate it for at least two hours until it is cold. 3. Finally, decorate with strawberries and serve.

Per Serving: Calories 131; Fat 6.76g; Sodium 20mg; Carbs 7.72g; Fiber 2.2g; Sugar 1.59g; Protein 12.27g

Nutty Apple Porridge

Prep time: 10 minutes | Cook time: 5 minutes | Servings: 4

Ingredients:

2 cups unsweetened almond milk	½ teaspoon organic vanilla extract
3 tablespoons walnuts, chopped	Pinch of ground cinnamon
3 tablespoons sunflower seeds	½ of a small apple, cored and sliced
2 large apples, peeled, cored and grated	1 small banana, peeled and sliced

Directions:

1. Mix milk, walnuts, sunflower seeds, grated apple, vanilla and cinnamon in a big pan and cook for 3-5 minutes on medium-low heat. 2. Then, transfer the porridge to serving bowls and add your preferred fruit on top before serving.

Per Serving: Calories 242; Fat 11.16g; Sodium 55mg; Carbs 32g; Fiber 5.1g; Sugar 23.09g; Protein 7.26g

Mixed Berries with Coconut Cream

Prep time: 10 minutes | Cook time: 0 minutes | Servings: 4

Ingredients:

2 (15-ounce) cans full-fat coconut milk	1-pint fresh blueberries
3 tablespoons agave	1-pint fresh raspberries
½ teaspoon vanilla extract	1-pint fresh strawberries, sliced

Directions:

1. To get ready for the recipe, chill the coconut milk in the refrigerator overnight. 2. After opening the can, scoop out the solid part and keep the liquid aside. 3. Mix agave and vanilla extract with the coconut solids in a bowl. Place the berries in four bowls and add the coconut cream on top. 4. It's best to serve right away.

Per Serving: Calories 468; Fat 19g; Sodium 1041mg; Carbs 53g; Fiber 8g; Sugar 26g; Protein 23g

Homemade Banana-Coconut Ice Cream

Prep time: 15 minutes | Cook time: 0 minutes | Servings: 6

Ingredients:

1 cup coconut cream	3 tbsp. honey extracted
½ cup Inverted sugar	¼ tsp cinnamon powder
2 large frozen bananas (chunks)	

Directions:

1. Whisk together coconut cream and inverted sugar in a bowl. 2. In another bowl, mix banana with honey and cinnamon. 3. Combine the two mixtures and stir well. Cover the bowl and refrigerate overnight. Stir the mixture 3 to 4 times to prevent it from crystallizing. 4. You can freeze it for 1 to 2 months.

Per Serving: Calories 237; Fat 14g; Sodium 3mg; Carbs 30g; Fiber 2.1g; Sugar 22.32g; Protein 1.98g

Butter Apple Pie

Prep time: 25 minutes | Cook time: 60 minutes | Servings: 12

Ingredients:

1 tbsp. fresh lemon juice

8 golden delicious apples, large, cored, peeled, diced into ⅛ inch slices

3 tbsp. potato starch

1 tsp ground cinnamon

¾ cup of white sugar

¼ tsp grated nutmeg, fresh

1 recipe pastry (for ten-inch double crust pie)

¼ cup unsalted butter, cold and diced into ¼-inch pieces

1 tbsp. white sugar

2 tsp milk

Directions:

1. To prepare the pie, preheat the oven to 425°F and place a baking stone on the lowest part of the oven. 2. Combine lemon juice, apple slices and milk in a large mixing bowl. 3. In another mixing bowl, combine ¾ cup sugar, potato starch, nutmeg, and cinnamon. 4. Roll out and dust half of the pie crust dough with flour and place it in a ten-inch pie pan. 5. Add half of the toppings and butter pieces, then sprinkle half of the potato starch mixture over it. 6. Fill the pan with remaining ingredients, sprinkle the remaining sweet mixture and buttery crumbs on top, then cover with the remaining pie crust dough. 7. Seal the edges, make a few holes with a fork, and brush with one tablespoon of sugar. 8. Place the pie on the baking stone in the preheated oven and reduce the temperature to 350°F. 9. Bake for approximately 60 minutes and check the edges halfway through. 10. Cool the pie for three hours on a wire rack before serving.

Per Serving: Calories 218; Fat 8.84g; Sodium 111mg; Carbs 35.72g; Fiber 3.4g; Sugar 19.54g; Protein 1.13g

Homemade Chocolate Pancakes

Prep time: 15 minutes | Cook time: 10 minutes | Servings: 12

Ingredients:

1¼ cups whole-grain flour

1 tablespoon baking powder

1 tablespoon ground flaxseed

1 tablespoon mini chocolate chips, vegan

2 tablespoons cocoa powder, unsweetened

¼ teaspoon of sea salt

1 tablespoon maple syrup

1 tablespoon apple cider vinegar

1 teaspoon vanilla extract, unsweetened

¼ cup applesauce, unsweetened

1 cup almond milk, unsweetened

Directions:

1. In a medium-sized bowl, combine whole-grain flour, flaxseed, baking powder, cocoa powder, salt, and chocolate chips by whisking them together. 2. In a separate small bowl, combine vinegar, maple syrup, vanilla, and almond milk by whisking them together. 3. Pour the milk mixture into the flour mixture and whisk until well combined. Allow the batter to rest for 10 minutes until it thickens and doubles in size. 4. Heat a large skillet over medium heat, spray it with oil, and pour one-twelfth of the batter into the pan. 5. Spread the batter gently and cook for 2 to 3 minutes until the bottom turns golden brown. 6. Flip the pancake and continue cooking for 2 minutes until done. 7. Transfer the pancake to a plate and repeat with the remaining batter. Serve immediately.

Per Serving: Calories 251; Fat 0.3g; Sodium 67mg; Carbs 3g; Fiber 5.7g; Sugar 7g; Protein 3.2g

Chocolate Banana Bread

Prep time: 15 minutes | Cook time: 1 hour | Servings: 15

Ingredients:

1 cup all-purpose flour	¼ cup almonds (thinly sliced)
1 tsp. salt	2 tsps. vanilla
½ cup whole wheat flour	3 medium mashed bananas
1 tsp. baking soda	1 tsp. cinnamon
¾ cup sugar	¼ cup mini dark chocolate chips
½ cup olive oil	

Directions:

1. First, preheat the oven to 325°F. 2. Then, mash the bananas in a small container. 3. In a large mixing bowl, mix together the sugar and olive oil until it becomes smooth. 4. Add the mashed banana and vanilla to the mixture and continue to mix. 5. In a medium-sized bowl, combine the flour, salt, baking soda, and cinnamon by whisking them together. 6. Add the flour mixture to the banana mixture and stir until it is well combined, even though it will be quite dense. 7. Next, mix in the almonds and chocolate chips. Grease an 8 x 4 or similar-sized loaf pan and spoon the batter into it. Bake at 350°F for about an hour and check it with a toothpick. 8. Once it's finished baking, let it cool for roughly fifteen minutes before taking it out of the pan.

Per Serving: Calories 153; Fat 7.58g; Sodium 242mg; Carbs 20.15g; Fiber 1.4g; Sugar 8g; Protein 1.68g

Although you may lose weight with the Body Reset diet, it's important to remember that the diet may not provide you with all the essential nutrients, particularly protein and healthy fats, especially during the program's first phase. Additionally, you may not feel like you're "eating more, exercising less," as the diet claims. In fact, you may feel like you're not eating much at all, while having to put in a lot of walking time. If you do decide to try the diet, it's important to make sure you're getting enough fiber, as recommended by Pasternak. Furthermore, the recipes and recommendations for "smoothies, stir-fries, scrambles, salads, and soups" could form the basis of a healthy eating plan going forward, even without the three-phased reset program.

It's worth remembering that following a long-term or short-term diet may not be necessary for you, and many diets out there simply don't work, particularly in the long term. While we don't endorse fad diets or unsustainable weight loss methods, we provide the facts so that you can make an informed decision that works best for your nutritional needs, genetic blueprint, budget, and goals. If your goal is weight loss, it's important to remember that losing weight isn't necessarily the same as being your healthiest self. There are many other ways to pursue health, including exercise, sleep, and other lifestyle factors that play a major role in your overall health. Ultimately, the best diet is always the one that is balanced and fits your lifestyle.

VOLUME EQUIVALENTS (DRY)

US STANDARD	METRIC (APPROXIMATE)
⅛ teaspoon	0.5 mL
¼ teaspoon	1 mL
½ teaspoon	2 mL
¾ teaspoon	4 mL
1 teaspoon	5 mL
1 tablespoon	15 mL
¼ cup	59 mL
½ cup	118 mL
¾ cup	177 mL
1 cup	235 mL
2 cups	475 mL
3 cups	700 mL
4 cups	1 L

VOLUME EQUIVALENTS (LIQUID)

US STANDARD	US STANDARD (OUNCES)	METRIC (APPROXIMATE)
2 tablespoons	1 fl.oz	30 mL
¼ cup	2 fl.oz	60 mL
½ cup	4 fl.oz	120 mL
1 cup	8 fl.oz	240 mL
1½ cup	12 fl.oz	355 mL
2 cups or 1 pint	16 fl.oz	475 mL
4 cups or 1 quart	32 fl.oz	1 L
1 gallon	128 fl.oz	4 L

TEMPERATURES EQUIVALENTS

FAHRENHEIT (F)	CELSIUS (C)(APPROXIMATE)
225 ℉	107℃
250 ℉	120℃
275 ℉	135℃
300 ℉	150℃
325 ℉	160℃
350 ℉	180℃
375 ℉	190℃
400 ℉	205℃
425 ℉	220℃
450 ℉	235℃
475 ℉	245℃
500 ℉	260℃

WEIGHT EQUIVALENTS

US STANDARD	METRIC (APPROXINATE)
1 ounce	28 g
2 ounces	57 g
5 ounces	142 g
10 ounces	284 g
15 ounces	425g
16 ounces (1 pound)	455 g
1.5pounds	680 g
2pounds	907g

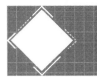

Appendix 2 Recipes Index

Made in the USA
Las Vegas, NV
21 November 2023

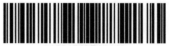